3

Revision for the MRCP Part 2

Data interpretation,
case histories and
photographic cases

WDRAWN

For Saunders

Commissioning Editor Laurence Hunter
Project Editor Sarah Keer-Keer
Project Controller Frances Affleck
Design direction Erik Bigland

Revision for the MRCP Part 2

Data interpretation, case histories and photographic cases

Debra King FRCP

Consultant Physician in Geriatric Medicine
Department of Medicine for the elderly
Wirral Hospital
Arrowe Park Road, Upton
Wirral, Merseyside

W. B. SAUNDERS

Edinburgh • London • New York • Philadelphia • Sydney • Toronto

W.B. SAUNDERS
An imprint of Harcourt Brace and Company Limited

© Harcourt Brace & Company Limited 1999

Ⓡ is a registered trade mark of Harcourt Brace and Company Limited

First published 1999

ISBN 0702022446

British Library Cataloguing in Publication Data
A catalogue record for this book is available from the British Library.

Library of Congress Cataloging in Publication Data
A catalog record for this book is available from the Library of Congress.

Medical knowledge is constantly changing. As new information becomes available, changes in treatment, procedures, equipment and the use of drugs become necessary. The authors and the publishers have, as far as it is possible, taken care to ensure that the information given in this text is accurate and up to date. However, readers are strongly advised to confirm that the information, especially with regard to drug usage, complies with current legislation and standards of practice.

Printed in China

Preface

There are many revision texts for MRCP part II. There is no substitute for adequate knowledge, which should be sought using reference texts but practising example questions is advantageous. This book contains examples of questions candidates will meet in the written section of the examination. There is discussion of all the questions. The photographic material section contains cases that may also be included in the short case section of the clinical examination. I am always heartened by the enthusiasm patients show in volunteering for clinical photographs to help doctors learn. There is always something to learn from each clinical case and experience and practice at examination technique will make the challenge of the MRCP part II examination easier for candidates. I hope this book will also make that challenge an easier one.

Acknowledgements

I would like to thank Mrs Susan Stewart for her patience, support and expert typing of the manuscript. I thank the patients all of whom were willing and most eager to be photographed to produce the clinical slides. It is always refreshing to note how patients want to help doctors learn and without their goodwill clinical texts and bedside teaching would not exist.

Contents

To study medicine without reading text books is like going to sea without charts, but to study medicine without dealing with patients is not to go to sea at all.

Sir William Osler (1849–1919). Professor of medicine, Oxford University.

William Osler was born in Canada and studied medicine in Montreal. He was a great advocate of clinical bedside teaching. He wrote widely on this as well as hereditary telangiectasia, lupus erythematosus and polycythaemia rubra vera. His name is linked with several conditions. Osler disease or Osler–Rendu–Weber disease or syndrome (hereditary haemorrhagic telangiectasia), Osler nodes (painful indurated areas on the pads of the fingers, which are sometimes seen in sub-acute bacterial endocarditis), Osler–Vaquez disease (polycythaemia rubra vera). He died of bronchopneumonia in 1919.

Introduction

The MRCP examination is under constant review and up-to-date details can be obtained from the Royal College of Physicians of London, 11 St Andrews Place, Regents Park, London NW1 4LE. The written examination consists of three sections: photographic material, data interpretation and case histories. The pass rate of the written examination is 75%; 60% will receive a clear pass and 15% a bare pass. The bare pass candidates can obtain an overall pass by making up marks in the clinical section. In the future once the written section has been passed it will not have to be repeated if a candidate fails the clinical section only (within a given time limit). There will therefore be a separation of the written and clinical sections of the part II examination. The number of attempts at MRCP part II will also be unlimited as opposed to the maximum of six attempts, which was imposed previously.

The written examination is set by a committee of examiners and questions are set several months in advance of the exam. The answers to each question are discussed, debated and finally agreed. Recent scientific developments that may occur between the setting of the question and the actual exam are taken into account when the papers are marked. Typical questions asked are: what is the most likely diagnosis?; what investigations (list two) would you request?; and what is the treatment? In the case history section in particular there is usually more than one answer as in real life, when we usually formulate a differential diagnosis. Marks are therefore given in a graded system with the maximum marks for the most likely diagnosis for example, but some marks can be gained for the less best but possible answer. In the data interpretation section it is more common that there is only one answer to the question. The number of marks available for each question is printed on the examination paper. Each question is marked by a team of examiners who will mark the same question to decrease inter-observer variation. Excessive replies will be ignored by examiners. Hence if a candidate is asked to give the two most important investigations to be requested and lists six the examiners will automatically delete the last four responses and mark the first two. In other words, they will not seek out the correct answers from multiple replies. The candidate's replies need to be specific and concise. This is all part of the examination technique. This can be improved with practice. Remember there are usually clues to the answers in the question although occasionally aspects are given to try and confuse the candidate, especially in the case histories and the candidate must give their best answer on the balance of probabilities. This is as in much the same way as a clinician comes to the most likely diagnosis based on the evidence gathered.

This book contains three sections: photographic material, data interpretation and case histories with questions, answers and explanations. Where possible clinical pointers are given as similar cases can be seen in the clinical section when discussion will be required with the examiners. Investigations, especially X-rays, ECGs and echocardiograms can also be produced alongside a short case or long case in the clinical exam and the candidate will be expected to interpret and discuss the investigations. Whilst this text is mainly directed to the written section, the cases described are also typical of those seen in the clinical examination.

Photographic cases

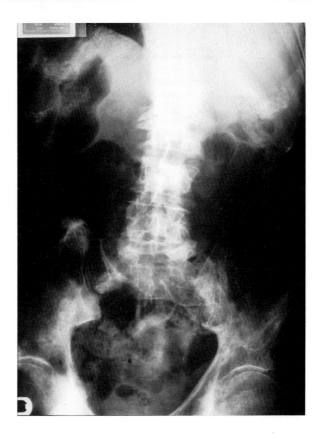

Questions

This 70-year-old man presented with pain on micturition and weakness in his legs causing frequent falls.

a. What does the X-ray show?
b. What is the cause of the X-ray changes?
c. Name two other symptoms he may have.
d. What is the most likely cause of his falls?

Answers

a. Multiple sclerotic metastases with areas of radiolucency.

b. Carcinoma of prostate metastasising to bone.

c. Symptoms of prostatic obstruction (frequency, hesitancy, nocturia, poor stream, urgency and terminal dribbling), bone pain (backache) or symptoms due to hypercalcaemia (polyuria, polydipsia, constipation, renal calculi and depression).

d. Spastic paraparesis due to spinal cord compression. The legs are weak and there may be diffuse atrophy. The tone and reflexes are increased and the plantar responses extensor. There will be a sensory level. This is a neurological emergency and requires urgent investigation (MRI – scan of spinal cord and/or myelogram) and treatment (surgical debulking of tumour and/or radiotherapy).

Discussion

Prostatic carcinoma is the most common malignancy in men over 65 years of age and 20% of cases of prostatic obstruction are due to carcinoma. The tumour may spread locally causing obstruction of one or both ureters or invasion of the rectum, resulting in stricture formation. Distant spread occurs via the bloodstream (which may be venous or arterial) particularly to the bones. The bones most frequently involved in descending order are: pelvis, vertebrae, upper femur, sternum and skull. Other tumours that metastasise to bone include: breast, bronchus, thyroid and kidney. Bony metastases from the prostate are usually 'sclerotic' or bone forming (osteoblastic) and there may be islands of radiolucency. Bone secondaries from a breast primary may be osteoblastic or osteolytic producing both areas of sclerosis and radiolucency on a plain X-ray. Other tumours metastasising to bone usually cause osteolytic areas. Osteoblastic metastases usually produce a raised alkaline phosphatase and the calcium may be low, normal or high. Osteolytic metastases are more likely to produce hypercalcaemia. Skeletal metastases from a primary prostatic carcinoma result in a raised serum acid phosphatase in 40% of cases, which is rarely raised by a primary tumour alone.

The usual clinical presentation of bone secondaries is bone pain, pathological fracture or symptoms and signs of hypercalcaemia. The prostate gland can be biopsied transrectally to confirm the diagnosis. Other investigations that will confirm the findings on the plain X-ray include radio-isotope bone scanning and bone biopsy (iliac crest). The bone marrow may sometimes be involved producing a pancytopenia when a bone marrow aspiration will confirm the diagnosis.

Treatment of bony metastases is symptomatic. Bone pain often responds to non-steroidal anti-inflammatory drugs and/or local radiotherapy. Pathological fractures are best treated by internal fixation to relieve pain and allow early mobilisation. Prostatic tumours have a fairly good prognosis when treated by hormonal manipulation, e.g. oestrogen, orchidectomy. It is also worth performing a prostatectomy if there are local symptoms.

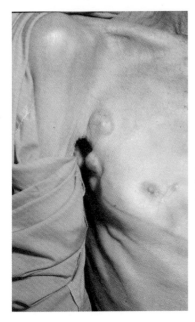
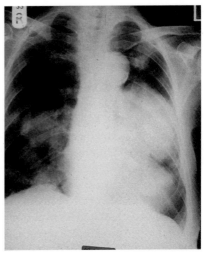

Questions

This man presented with backache 3 months previously. His blood pressure was 200/110 and his haemoglobin was 19.5 g/dl.

a. What are the abnormalities shown?
b. What is the underlying diagnosis?
c. What is the reason for his haemoglobin level?

Answers

a. Skin and lung metastases.

b. Adenocarcinoma of the kidney (hypernephroma or Grawitz tumour).

c. Polycythaemia caused by increased erythropoietin production by the tumour.

Discussion

Other tumours that may metastasise to the lung and skin include lung, breast, stomach and uterine tumours. Adenocarcinoma of the kidney is more common in males and the incidence increases with age. It usually arises from the upper pole of the kidney and is bilateral in 5% of cases. Blood-born spread can occur to lung and skin and lymphatic spread occurs to liver and bone. Local spread may cause vena caval obstruction or a left-sided varicoele if there is spread into the left renal vein into which the testicular veins drain.

A hypernephroma most commonly presents as painless haematuria and pain and/or a palpable mass in the loin. It may also cause pyrexia, anaemia (normochromic/normocytic or hypochromic/microcytic if there is haematuria) and a raised ESR. Hypercalcaemia may be due to bone metastases or secretion of a parathyroid hormone-like substance by the tumour. Cushing's syndrome is produced by adrenocorticotrophic hormone (ACTH) production and polycythaemia by erythropoietin production by the tumour. The patient is often hypertensive as in this case. Neurological abnormalities due to cerebral metastases and other phenomenon (peripheral neuropathy) can occur. If the tumour is particularly vascular, high output cardiac failure may be the presenting feature.

The diagnosis is almost always made on intravenous urography. A CT scan should also be undertaken to discover any evidence of local spread and the exact nature of the tumour. Nephrectomy is the treatment of choice even if there are distant metastases as these later regress. Local lymphatic spread is associated with a particularly poor prognosis. The tumour is not responsive to chemotherapy or radiotherapy but patients with painful metastases may improve with medroxyprogesterone acetate (Provera). The survival rate is 50% at 5 years and 30% at 10 years.

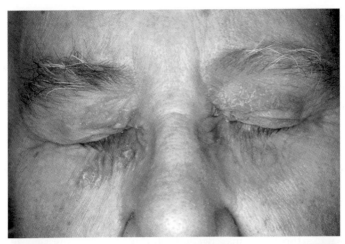

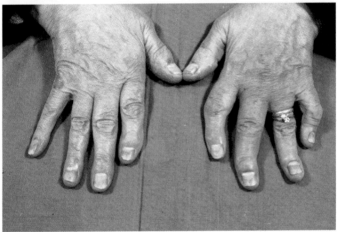

Questions

This woman complained of intermittent episodes of bloody diarrhoea for 20 years.

a. Name two abnormalities in her hands.
b. What is the skin lesion?
c. What is the most likely cause of her diarrhoea?

Answers

a. Boutonnière deformity on left little finger, subluxation and swelling of left index finger proximal interphalangeal joint, and subluxation of left middle finger distal interphalangeal joint. There is also extensive onycholysis (detachment of the nail from the nail bed).

b. Psoriasis around the eyes and also at the base of the right little finger.

c. Inflammatory bowel disease (ulcerative colitis, *Crohn's disease). Inflammatory bowel disease is more common in patients with psoriasis and is associated with *HLA-B27*. The long intermittent history in this case makes colonic tumour unlikely, which should be considered at presentation.

Discussion

Psoriatic arthropathy may occur in the absence of any skin lesions. Onycholysis occurs in 80% of cases. Other nail changes include: pitting, hyperkeratosis and ridging. The disease is inherited (30% of patients give a family history) but there is no †Mendelian pattern, more a multifactorial inheritance. *HLA-B13* and *B17* are more common in patients with psoriasis as is *HLA-B27*. The latter is especially more common in those with sacroiliac involvement.

The arthritis has similarities to rheumatoid arthritis and it may affect any joint in the body. Unlike rheumatoid arthritis it is asymmetrical and also affects the distal interphalangeal joints and the sacroiliac joints. The sacroiliac joints are affected radiographically in 20% of all cases and ankylosing spondylitis occurs more frequently than in the general population. Rheumatoid factor is absent from the serum in psoriatic arthritis, hence the term 'sero-negative spondoarthritides', which includes: psoriatic arthritis, ankylosing spondylitis, enteropathic enteritis (occurs in 15% of cases) and ‡Reiter's syndrome. Psoriatic arthritis has a broad spectrum of severity including an extensive deforming arthritis with ankylosis and dissolution of bones (*arthritis mutilans*), which is usually accompanied by sacroiliitis. Arthritis mutilans is less painful than it looks and this is thought to be due to nerve damage.

Treatment is similar for patients with rheumatoid arthritis: non-steroidal anti-inflammatory drugs, steroids, sulphasalazine, gold etc. Anti-malarial drugs such as chloroquine and hydroxychloroquine should be avoided as they cause exfoliation.

The prognosis is better overall than cases of rheumatoid arthritis.

---

*B.B. Crohn (born 1884), American physician.

†G. Mendel (1822–1884), Austrian monk and botanist.

‡H.C. Reiter (1881–1969), German professor of hygiene.

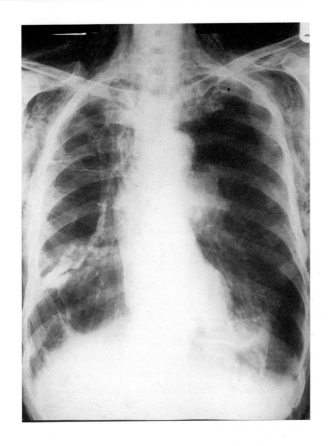

Question

List three abnormalities on this chest X-ray.

Answers

1. Right pleural calcification
2. Left basal pneumothorax
3. Subcutaneous (surgical) emphysema.

Discussion

Pleural calcification is a sign of previous exposure to asbestos. Pleural plaques also occur, which are calcified linear areas often seen on the diaphragmatic pleura. These features are harmless. Extensive pleural calcification can also occur after a haemothorax.

The most common type of pneumothorax is 'spontaneous' and occurs usually in young, healthy males. The source is an air leak from a tiny bleb on the lung surface. About 20% of spontaneous pneumothoraces occur within the first year. A pneumothorax may occur secondary to other diseases: chronic bronchitis, asthma, lung abscess, bronchial carcinoma, trauma, pulmonary fibrosis and tuberculosis. The patient presents with sudden onset of breathlessness and chest pain, which is usually pleuritic. In a small number of cases the pneumothorax may be under tension when the communication between the lungs and pleural space is a one-way valve from lung to pleural space. The mediastinum is pushed to the opposite side with compromise of the remaining lung. Circulatory failure may result. This is a medical emergency and requires an urgent chest drain. Only small, asymptomatic pneumothoraces should be managed conservatively. Most require an intercostal chest drain, which is usually positioned in the second intercostal space in the mid-clavicular line or the fifth intercostal space in the mid-axillary line and then connected to an underwater seal drain. The drain bubbles and when it stops it signifies expansion of the lung, which is confirmed by a chest X-ray and then the tube can be removed. If the bubbling is persistent, then further intervention is required: pleurodesis (surgical or chemical) or thoracotomy with oversewing of the lung perforation. Subcutaneous emphysema in this case occurred due to leakage of air from the intercostal tube, which has been removed. This is the most common cause of subcutaneous emphysema. Other causes include: severe asthma, trauma, intermittent positive pressure ventilation and a ruptured oesophagus.

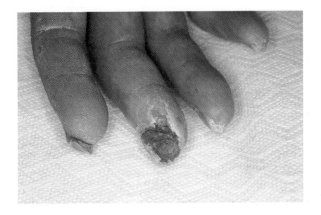

Questions

This 80-year-old woman had difficulty swallowing.

a. What does this X-ray show and what is the cause?
b. Name two other causes of this condition.
c. List two possible causes of her symptom.
d. What is the underlying diagnosis in this case?

Answers

a. Necrotic areas on the index and middle fingers and dystrophic changes on the remaining fingers due to severe *Raynaud's phenomenon.

b. Systemic lupus erythematosus (SLE), rheumatoid arthritis, polymyositis, idiopathic hypothyroidism, cervical rib and systemic sclerosis.

c. Oesophageal immotility and oesophageal stricture.

d. Systemic sclerosis.

Discussion

Systemic sclerosis is mainly a disease of middle-aged women with involvement of the following systems:

1. **Locomotor** – polyarthralgia (may be indistinguishable from rheumatoid arthritis), polymyositis.

2. **Skin** – Raynaud's phenomenon, sclerodactyly, telangectasia, tight smooth waxy pigmented skin (50%), skin ulcers (40%), vitiligo, subcutaneous calcification (10%).

3. **Heart** – cardiomyopathy, pericardial effusion, hypertension (malignant and may be fatal).

4. **Lungs** – fibrosis, aspiration pneumonia.

5. **Gut** – dysphagia (70%) due to immobility and peptic strictures, hiatus hernia, dilated second part of duodenum and diverticulae, colonic diverticulae may rupture and cause diarrhoea and constipation (although rare), malabsorption due to decreased small bowel motility and bacterial overgrowth.

6. **Renal** – progressive renal failure (common cause of death).

7. **Neurological** – (rare) unilateral trigeminal neuropathy.

There are overlap syndromes: Crest syndrome, Thibierge–Weissenbach syndrome (subcutaneous calcification and acrosclerosis), morphoea (isolated skin lesions that rarely progress to systemic sclerosis), mixed connective tissue disease (overlap with systemic sclerosis, SLE and dermatomyositis). Treatment is usually symptomatic and the overall 5-year survival is 70%. Patients with Crest syndrome and morphoea have a better prognosis. Poor prognostic features include older age at presentation and evidence of cardiac, pulmonary or renal involvement.

---

*M. Raynaud (1834–1881), French physician.

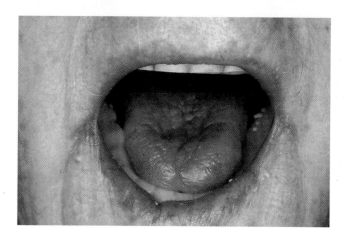

Questions

This 75-year-old woman complained of breathlessness on exertion and diarrhoea.

a. Name two abnormalities.
b. What is the diagnosis?
c. What is the most likely cause?
d. List two other symptoms she may have.

Answers

a. Glossitis and angular stomatitis

b. Iron deficiency anaemia

c. Colonic carcinoma

d. Palpitations and tiredness (caused by anaemia), weight loss, constipation, rectal bleeding and abdominal pain (caused by colonic carcinoma).

Discussion

Glossitis is a sign of anaemia due to iron, B_{12} or folate deficiency. Angular stomatitis is usually associated with iron deficiency anaemia. The patient has pale conjunctivae and may have brittle nails or koilonychia in severe cases. The blood films show microcytic, hypochromic red cells due to chronic iron deficiency anaemia secondary to chronic blood loss. Colonic carcinomas, particularly caecal, may present with anaemia and its symptoms (occult carcinoma), many months before gastrointestinal symptoms occur. In this situation it is essential to take a full history including dietary history (older people have a poor dietary intake of iron) as well as family history (colonic carcinoma, pernicious anaemia, peptic ulcers), past medical history, (gastrectomy – B_{12} and iron deficiency) and ask for evidence of blood loss (nosebleeds, haematuria, rectal bleeding and menstruation). If no underlying cause of iron deficiency anaemia is apparent from the history or examination, then sigmoidoscopy and barium enema should be performed in the first instance. The cause of anaemia should always be established.

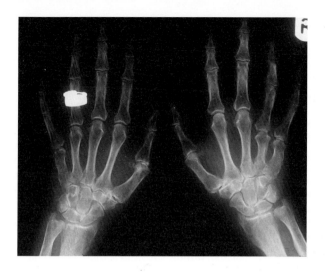

Questions

This childless woman complained of headaches. Her blood pressure was 200/100.

a. What abnormalities can be seen?
b. What is the diagnosis?
c. What is the most likely cause of her hypertension?
d. Name two other causes of this X-ray finding.

Answers

a. Short fourth and fifth metacarpals, especially on the right hand.
b. *Turner's syndrome.
c. Coarctation of the aorta.
d. Pseudohypoparathyroidism and Noonan's syndrome.

Discussion

Turner's syndrome is characterised by ovarian disgenesis with a 45XO karyotype. Patients often present with primary amenorrhoea and are sterile (as in this case). The patient is short in stature, has a short, webbed neck, an increased carrying angle, widely spaced nipples and absent secondary sexual characteristics (unless treated with oestrogens). As well as short metacarpals the nails are often hypoplastic. Other features include: low hairline, double eye lashes, high arched palate, café au lait spots and black naevi, mental retardation (10%), ptosis and intestinal telangectasia. There is an increased incidence of diabetes mellitus and †Hashimoto's thyroiditis. Cardiovascular defects occur in 20% of cases: coarctation of the aorta, VSD, ASD, aortic stenosis.

Noonan's syndrome has a similar phenotype to Turner but a normal 46XX karyotype. The patient is fertile and more likely to have right-sided heart lesions (pulmonary stenosis).

Pseudohypoparathyroidism is an inherited disorder resulting in a peripheral resistance to parathyroid hormone (PTH). There is hypocalcaemia, hyperphosphataemia and a raised PTH level. Patients often have short stature, mental retardation, obesity and a moon face. There is calcification of the basal ganglia on the skull X-ray and an increased incidence of cutaneous moniliasis.

---

*H.H. Turner (born 1892). American physician.
†H. Hashimoto (1881–1934). Japanese surgeon.

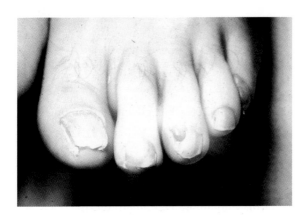

Questions

This 16-year-old boy presented with epilepsy as did his brother.

a. What abnormality can be seen?
b. What is the diagnosis?
c. What is the inheritance?
d. What may be seen on fundoscopy?

Answers

a. There are subungual fibromas on the third and little toes.
b. Tuberous sclerosis also known as epiloia, *Bourneville disease and Pringle disease.
c. Autosomal dominant.
d. Retinal phakomas (discrete white gliomatous tumours).

Discussion

Tuberous sclerosis is characterised by a triad of epilepsy, mental retardation and adenoma sebaceum. The latter are reddish nodules, which are angiofibromas, developing in childhood on the face (cheeks and nasolabial folds). The prevalence of the condition is 5/100 000. There is no treatment other than the control of epilepsy. Clinical features can be categorised as follows:

1. **Skin** – shagreen patches (circumscribed areas of sub-epidermal fibrosis occurring in the lumbosacral region), cafe au lait spots, subungual fibromas, adenoma sebaceum, amelanotic naevi (ovoid depigmented patches on trunk and limbs, which look like the leaf of the mountain ash – 'ash leaf hypomelanosis' – and are frequently present at birth).

2. **Eyes** – retinal phakomas.

3. **Neurological** – mental retardation, epilepsy, cortical tubers (firm white areas containing astrocytes and broadening cortical gyri), gliomas, subependymal nodules.

4. **Skeletal** – bone cysts.

5. **Other organs** – cardiac rabdomyomas, lung and kidney hamartomas. There is an association with polycystic kidneys and endocrine tumours are more common.

---

*D.M. Bourneville (1840–1909). French neurologist.

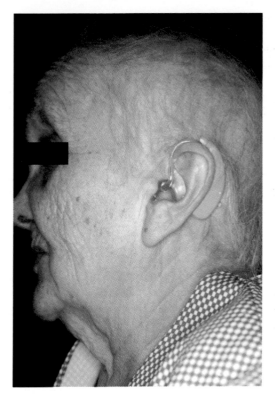 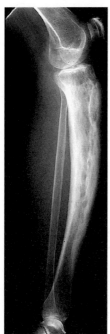

Questions

This woman complained of pain in her leg.

a. What is the diagnosis?
b. Give two reasons for her deafness.
c. Give two possible causes for the pain in her leg.
d. List two biochemical abnormalities.

Answers

a. *Paget's disease of bone (skull and tibia with anterior bowing in this case).

b. Pagetic involvement of the ear ossicles and compression of the 8th cranial nerve due to narrowing of its foramina due to skull bone overgrowth.

c. Obvious deformity (anterior bowing of tibia) and pathological fracture.

d. Raised serum alkaline phosphatase and 24-hour urinary hydroxyproline level, which are used to measure the severity of disease and its monitoring. Hypercalcaemia may occur if the patient is immobile.

Discussion

Paget's disease is more common in males, affects 1% of the population over the age of 50 years and has a familial incidence. There is increased bone resorption and deposition of abnormal bone (*osteitis deformans*) resulting in thickening, deformity and pathological fractures. The bones of the axial skeleton and limbs are more commonly involved. The skull enlarges due to thickening and there may be large areas of resorption (*osteoporosis circumscripta*).

Other features include:

1. Basilar invagination causing brainstem symptoms and signs.
2. Spinal stenosis causing spastic paraparesis and kyphosis.
3. High output cardiac failure.
4. Optic atrophy and angioid streaks in the retina.
5. Osteoarthrosis of related joints.
6. Urolithiasis, constipation and depression (resulting from hypercalcaemia).
7. Sarcomatous change (< 1% of cases).

Treatment is symptomatic. Specific drugs used to contain the disease include biphosphonates and calcitonin.

---

*Sir James Paget (1814–1899). British surgeon

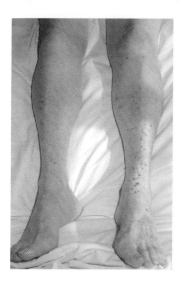

Questions

This 35-year-old woman complained of generalised aches and pains and pleuritic central chest pain. She also had a rash on the dorsum of her hands and complained of feeling depressed.

a. What is shown on this slide?
b. Name two possible causes of her chest pain.
c. What is the underlying condition?
d. Name two drugs that may be implicated in this condition.

Answers

a. Vasculitic rash.

b. Pleurisy, pericarditis.

c. Systemic lupus erythematosus (SLE).

d. Hydralazine (slow acetylators), procainamide (rapid acetylators), primidone, phenytoin, isoniazid, chlorpromazine. The condition is reversed by withdrawal of these drugs and neurological and renal involvement is rare.

Discussion

SLE is a multi-system disorder that is more common in women (9:1) (Discoid LE if only the skin is involved, female to male 2:1). There is a hereditary component to its aetiology and an association with *HLA-D3*. The disease affects the small arterioles and capillaries and circulating immune complexes are widely deposited.

Clinical features can be categorised as follows:

1. **Skin** – vasculitis is the most common rash. Non-specific erythema may occur as well as a malar flush ('butterfly' rash) (50%), alopecia (60%) photosensitivity (backs of hands as in this case), oral ulcerations and nail fold infarcts (10%), telangectasia and Raynaud's phenomenon (10%).

2. **Renal** – nephrotic syndrome, nephritis and hypertension (50%).

3. **Locomotor** – symmetrical polyarthralgia similar to rheumatoid arthritis rarely erosive or deforming. Deformity may occur due to tendon contracture (Jaccoud's arthritis).

4. **Neurological** – neuro-psychiatric symptoms, especially depression, is common (70%). Chorea, myelitis, epilepsy and peripheral neuropathy.

5. **Lungs** – pleurisy, pleural effusion, patchy consolidation and reticulonodular shadows on the chest X-ray, fibrosis.

6. **Heart** – pericarditis (30%), cardiomyopathy, non-bacterial endocarditis of aortic and mitral valves (*†Libman–Sacks), conductive defects (rare).

7. **Haematology** – raised ESR (90%), thrombocytopenia (30%), anaemia (normochromic/normocytic or haemolytic), leucopenia, hepatosplenomegaly (15%), lymphadenopathy (15%), anti-DNA

(double stranded) antibodies are specific for SLE, serum complement level (especially C4) is low.

Treatment is only required in relapses and includes: non-steroidal anti-inflammatory drugs, anti-malarials, steroids, azathioprine. The 10-year survival rate is 90%.

Other causes of vasculitis include:

- Polyarteritis nodosa
- Rheumatoid arthritis
- ‡Wegener's granulomatosis
- Systemic sclerosis
- Septicaemia
- Drugs
- Infective endocarditis
- §‖Henoch–Schönlein purpura.

*E. Libman (1872–1946). American physician.
†B. Sacks (1873–1939). American physician.
‡F. Wegener (born 1907). German pathologist.
§E.H. Henoch (1820–1910). German paediatrician.
‖J.L. Schönlein (1793–1864). German physician.

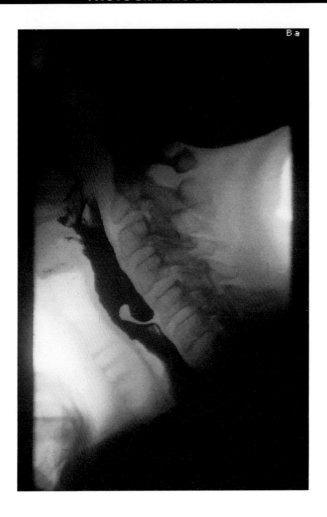

Questions

a. What type of X-ray is this?
b. What does it show?
c. Name one symptom the patient may have.

Answers

a. Barium swallow.
b. A pharyngeal pouch.
c. Dysphagia, regurgitation of food, symptoms due to aspiration pneumonitis.

Discussion

A pharyngeal pouch is more common in elderly men. It is a mucosal protrusion between the thyropharyngeous and cricopharyngeous muscles. It develops posteriorly in the weakest area (Killian's dehiscence) and moves laterally when it grows (usually to the left side). Treatment is by surgical excision and myotomy of the cricopharyngeous muscle.

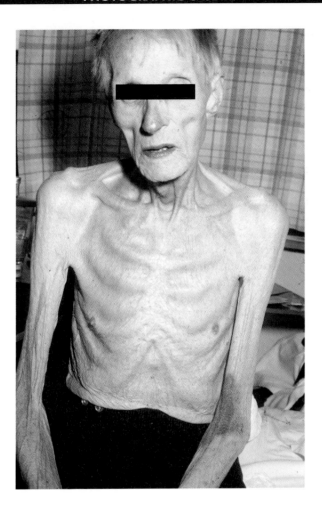

Questions

This 80-year-old man had an episode of chorea as a child. He is currently taking digoxin 250 mcg o.d. and frusemide 250 mg o.d. He presented with recurrent falls.

a. What is the physical sign?
b. What is a possible cause of this?
c. What is the underlying cardiovascular diagnosis?

Answers

a. Cachexia.

b. Cardiac cachexia (multifactorial aetiology – see later, digoxin toxicity).

c. Rheumatic mitral valve disease.

Discussion

This patient had *Sydenham's chorea as a child. This is an infectious chorea (St Vitus' dance) causing chorea (20% unilateral), emotional and behavioural problems. It occurs between 5 and 15 years of age and is more common in girls (2:1). In 30% of cases it occurs up to 3 months after rheumatic fever (due to group A streptococci). One-third of cases show cardiac involvement at presentation and a further third develop chronic rheumatic heart disease. Sydenham's chorea can also occur in pregnancy and in women taking the oral contraceptive pill.

This patient has been treated with digoxin and diuretics for atrial fibrillation and congestive heart failure caused by rheumatic valvular heart disease. He is on a large dose of digoxin and could have lost weight due to toxicity (anorexia, nausea, vomiting, arrhythmias, xanthopsia). Cardiac cachexia is weight loss occurring as a consequence of chronic congestive heart failure. The aetiology is multi-factorial and includes: malabsorption, increased basal metabolic rate, anorexia and early satiety due to a congested liver pressing on the stomach. Cardiac cachexia occurs in up to 50% of patients with heart failure and is associated with increased morbidity and mortality. It is an underrecognised condition. The overall mortality in congestive heart failure is 50% at 5 years but in severe cases may be as high at 60% in the first year.

---

*T. Sydenham (1624–1689). British physician.

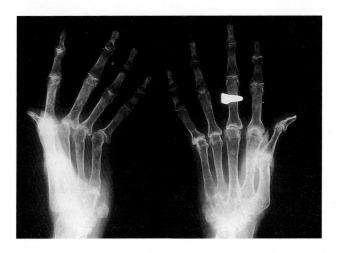

Questions

This patient complained of pain and tingling in his hands, especially at night.

a. What is the diagnosis?
b. What is the cause in this case?
c. Name two other causes of this condition.
d. What is the treatment?

Answers

a. Bilateral carpal tunnel syndrome.

b. Rheumatoid arthritis (subluxation of the metacarpo-phalangeal joints on the left).

c. Acromegaly, hypothyroidism, idiopathic (usually middle-aged, obese females), gout, osteoarthrosis of the wrist, pregnancy and the oral contraceptive pill.

d. Intracarpal steroid tunnel injection or surgical carpal tunnel decompression.

Discussion

Carpal tunnel syndrome causes pain, numbness or paraesthesia over the area supplied by the median nerve (palmar aspect of the first three-and-a-half fingers and tips of the first three-and-a-half fingers on the dorsum). The symptoms are worse at night. There may be wasting of the thenar eminence and weakness of thumb abduction, opposition and flexion. *Tinel's sign may be positive (percussion of the nerve produces tingling in its distribution) as may Phalen's sign (flexion of the wrist causes tingling). The diagnosis can be confirmed by nerve conduction studies but it is usually obvious clinically.

---

*J. Tinel (1879–1952). French neurologist.

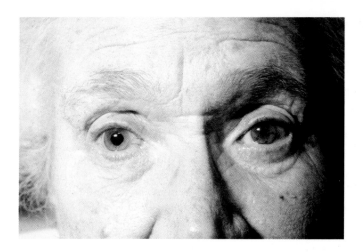

Questions

This woman had normal eye movements.

a. What is the abnormality?
b. Name an abnormal sign in her legs.
c. What is the diagnosis?
d. What is the treatment?

Answers

a. A mydriatic (dilated) right pupil.
b. Absent or diminished tendon reflexes.
c. *†Holmes–Adie pupil.
d. None.

Discussion

This is the most common cause of pupillary inequality (anisocoria), more minor degrees of which can be seen in up to 20% of the population. The tonic pupil reacts slowly to light and accommodation – convergence. There is denervation and super-sensitivity of the iris sphincter, which acts intensely to pupil constrictors and normally to pupil dilators. The lesion is thought to be in the ciliary ganglion. The iris may have vermiform movements at its borders and tendon reflexes are diminished or lost. The condition is almost always unilateral and chronic. It can occur acutely when there may be photophobia and blurring of vision. This must be distinguished from the ‡Argyll Robertson pupil, which is almost always bilateral. This is a small irregular pupil with an atrophic iris and an absent or reduced light response, and a preserved accommodation-convergence response. Argyll Robertson pupils occur in neurosyphilis but can rarely be present in diabetes mellitus. The lesion is thought to be in the mid-brain.

---

*Sir G.M. Holmes (1876–1965). British neurologist.
†W.J. Adie (1886–1935). British physician.
‡D.M.C.L. Argyll Robertson (1837–1909). British physician and ophthalmic surgeon.

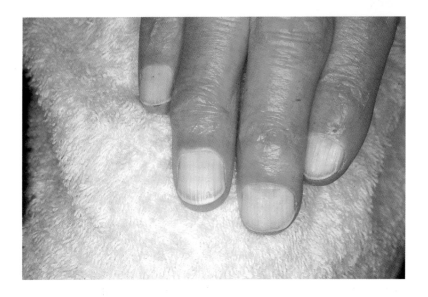

Questions

This 60-year-old man had a massive haematemesis.

a. What is the physical sign?
b. What is the underlying diagnosis?
c. What is the cause of his haematemesis?

Answers

a. Leuconychia due to chronic liver disease (hypoalbuminaemia).
b. Liver cirrhosis.
c. Oesophageal varices.

Discussion

A 'massive haematemesis' is indicative of varices but could be due to a duodenal ulcer, which is also more common in alcoholics. Alcoholism is the most common cause of cirrhosis and liver failure in the UK. Varices occur at sites of portacaval anastomoses when there is portal hypertension: oesophagus, lower third of rectum, umbilicus (caput medusae), sub-diaphragmatic and retro-peritoneal areas. Other signs of chronic liver disease are: jaundice, pigmentation, finger clubbing, palmar erythema, *Dupuytren's contracture, gynaecomastia, hepatosplenomegaly, ascites, testicular atrophy, purpura, spider naevi, flapping tremor and pallor.

Other causes of liver cirrhosis include

1. Chronic active hepatitis (lupoid hepatitis) – more common in females and associated with inflammatory bowel disease, diabetes mellitus, pulmonary fibrosis, thyroid disease, smooth muscle antibodies (60%), LE cells (15%), ANF (20–70%). This condition is steroid responsive.

2. Haemochromatosis (slate grey skin, diabetes, more common in males).

3. Viral (hepatitis B and C).

4. Cryptogenic.

5. †Wilson's disease (hepatolenticular degeneration).

6. Biliary obstruction.

7. Cardiac failure.

8. Constrictive pericarditis.

9. Drugs (methotrexate, isoniazid).

---

*Baron G. Dupuytren (1777–1895). French surgeon.
†S.A.K. Wilson (1877–1937). British neurologist.

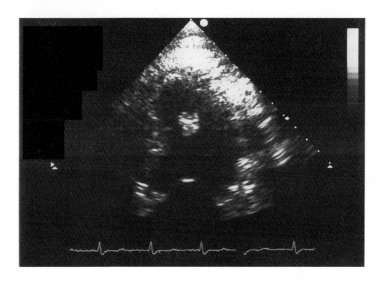

Questions

This 78-year-old man complained of sudden onset of pain in his right leg.

a. What is this investigation?
b. What does it show?
c. What is the most likely cause?
d. What is the cause of his symptoms?
e. What is the treatment?
f. Name two possible abnormalities on his ECG.

Answers

a. 2D (two-dimensional) echocardiogram.

b. Left ventricular apical aneurysm and organised thrombus.

c. Myocardial infarction.

d. Right femoral embolus.

e. Right femoral embolectomy. Lifelong anti-coagulation. Cardiac surgical intervention depends upon complications of the aneurysm and the operative risk of the patient.

f. Old myocardial infarction. Persistent ST elevation on an ECG is a feature of a left ventricular aneurysm.

Discussion

Left ventricular aneurysms are always the consequence of transmural myocardial infarctions and 50% will contain a thrombus. Spontaneous embolism can occur resulting in femoral occlusion, stroke and mesenteric vascular occlusion. The latter presents with colicky abdominal pain and bloody diarrhoea. When the aneurysm becomes large enough it may impair left ventricular function and cause cardiac failure. Complications include: angina, ventricular arrhythmias and rupture (rare). Clinically the patient has a double apical impulse and may have signs of left ventricular failure. The blood pressure is normal or low.

In selected patients left ventricular aneurectomy and coronary artery bypass grafting may be necessary. If surgery is contraindicated the patient should be managed conservatively, i.e. with frusemide and angiotensin-converting enzyme (ACE) inhibitors for heart failure and anti-arrhythmic drugs (amiodarone) for ventricular arrhythmias and lifelong warfarin. Symptomatic aneurysms have a poor prognosis and a 5-year survival rate of 20%.

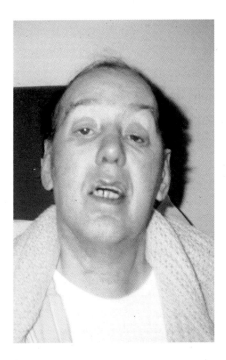

Questions

This man presented with polyuria and a painless foot ulcer.

a. What abnormalities can be seen? (name two)
b. What is the diagnosis?
c. What is its inheritance?
d. What is the cause of his symptoms?

Answers

a. Bilateral ptosis, transverse smile, frontal balding.

b. Dystrophia myotonica.

c. Autosomal dominant.

d. Diabetes mellitus (neuropathic ulcer). People with dystrophia myotonica have an increased incidence of diabetes mellitus.

Discussion

Dystrophia myotonica is more common in males and its features may become more pronounced in successive generations ('anticipation'). The patient has myopic facies, wasting of the facial muscles, ptosis, frontal balding and cataracts. If the arms are involved the reflexes are absent. Myotonia (delayed relaxation) is exacerbated by cold and excitement. The following factors are associated: cardiomyopathy (congestive heart failure and fatal arrhythmias, low blood pressure), impaired intellect and personality, nodular thyroid enlargement, testicular atrophy (reduced fertility), diabetes mellitus, dysphagia, hypoventilation. These subjects are an anaesthetic risk due to postoperative respiratory failure. There is no treatment for the weakness, which is a prominent feature but myotonia may be relieved by phenytoin, quinine or procainamide.

Myotonia congenita (*Thomsen's disease) is inherited as an autosomal dominant condition. There is myotonia but no other features of dystrophia myotonica, and reflexes are normal.

---

*A.J.T. Thomsen (1815–1896). Danish physician.

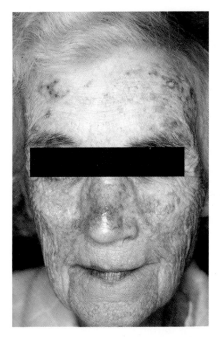

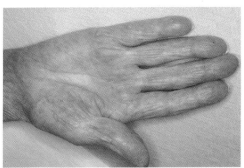

Questions

This patient had a 40-year history of ulcerative colitis.

a. What clinical features are present? (name two)
b. What is the diagnosis?
c. Which HLA associations are there? (list three)

Answers

a. Telangectasia, icterus, palmar erythema.
b. Chronic active hepatitis (lupoid hepatitis).
c. *HLA-A1, -B8, -DW3.*

Discussion

The signs are of chronic liver disease (see case 15). Chronic active hepatitis may follow hepatitis B or C, alcoholic hepatitis and is caused by some drugs (methyldopa, isoniazid). It is more common in women aged 15–50 years and may mimic acute viral hepatitis at the onset. There is peri-portal infiltration and piecemeal necrosis and fibrosis. Progression to cirrhosis is usual. This is a multi-system disorder and there may be fever, rashes, arthralgia, lymphadenopathy, pleurisy, pericarditis, pulmonary fibrosis, Coombs' positive haemolytic anaemia and thrombocytopenia. There is an association with thyroid disease, diabetes mellitus and inflammatory bowel disease (as in this case). Smooth muscle antibodies are present in 60% of cases, LE cells in 15% of cases and antinuclear factor in 20–70% of cases. The condition responds to steroids. Death may result from steroid complications, hepatic failure secondary to cirrhosis or gastrointestinal bleeding secondary to oesophageal varices.

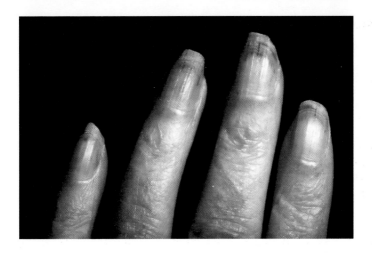

Questions

This patient with *†Ehlers–Danlos syndrome presented with pyrexia of unknown origin.

a. What is the clinical sign shown?
b. Name two causes of this sign.
c. What is the most likely cause in this case?
d. What is the underlying reason?

---

*E. Ehlers (1863–1937), Danish dermatologist.
†H.A. Danlos (1844–1912), French dermatologist.

Answers

a. Extensive splinter haemorrhages.

b. Trauma, connective tissue disease (rheumatoid arthritis, SLE, systemic sclerosis), subacute bacterial endocarditis (SABE).

c. SABE.

d. Mitral valve prolapse (MVP).

Discussion

In Ehlers–Danlos syndrome there is defective collagen giving a variety of symptoms and signs. There are eight types with different levels of severity and different inheritance patterns (dominant, recessive, X-linked). Symptoms include: hyperextensile joints and skin, myopia, kyphoscoliosis, purpura and poor healing skin. Complications include: spontaneous pneumothorax, MVP, recurrent joint dislocations, gastrointestinal bleeding and dissecting aneurysms. Subjects with significant MVP (audible mitral regurgitant murmur) should receive endocarditis antibiotic prophylaxis before dental procedures, upper respiratory tract surgery, sclerotherapy for oesophageal varices, oesophageal dilatation, surgery/instrumentation of lower bowel, gallbladder or genitourinary tract surgery and obstetric and gynaecological procedures. The usual regime is 3 g amoxycillin orally 1 h pre-operatively and for those with penicillin allergy, clindamycin 0.6 g orally 1 h pre-operatively. High-risk patients (those with prosthetic valves or previous endocarditis) should receive amoxycillin 1 g i.v. and gentamicin 120 mg i.v. pre-operatively, and amoxycillin 0.5 g orally 6 h postoperatively. Those with penicillin allergy should receive vancomycin 1 g i.v. over 1 h and gentamicin 120 mg i.v. pre-operatively.

Other signs of SABE include: finger clubbing, *Osler's nodes (painful indurated lesions in the finger pulps), †Janeway's lesions (red eruptions on the palms and soles that fade away like a bruise), fever, pallor, splenomegaly, microscopic haematuria (glomerulonephritis), café au lait spots (rare and late sign) and ‡Roth spots (oval retinal haemorrhage with pale centre also seen in SLE).

If SABE is suspected at least six blood cultures should be taken before i.v. benzylpenicillin and gentamicin are commenced. These antibiotics are continued until further microbiological data is available.

---

*Sir W. Osler (1849–1919), Canadian professor of medicine.
†E.G. Janeway (1841-1911), American physician.
‡M. Roth (1839–1914), Swiss pathologist.

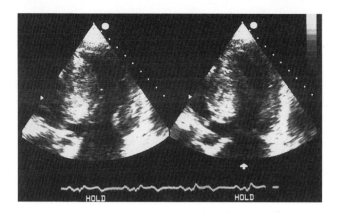

Questions

This patient complained of blackouts.

a. What is the abnormality in this 2D echocardiogram?
b. Give two possible reasons for blackouts.
c. What is the diagnosis?
d. What is the treatment?

Answers

a. Gross asymmetrical septal hypertrophy and a narrow left ventricular cavity.

b. Outflow obstruction, arrhythmias (there is an association with Wolff–Parkinson–White syndrome, which predisposes to atrial fibrillation that may lead to ventricular fibrillation).

c. Hypertrophic obstructive cardiomyopathy (HOCM).

d. Nitrates and diuretics should be avoided. Outflow obstruction is helped by beta blockade and calcium antagonists. Digoxin should only be prescribed if the patient is in atrial fibrillation. Amiodarone is used for ventricular arrhythmias.

Discussion

HOCM was only described as recently as 1958 by the pathologist Donald Teare. It is defined as 'an idiopathic heart muscle condition characterised by hypertrophied and non-dilated left and/or right ventricle(s) in the absence of a cardiac cause'. There is usually asymmetrical septal hypertrophy (ASH), systolic anterior movement of the mitral valve apparatus (SAM) and a small left ventricular cavity with a hypercontractile posterior wall. The mitral valve becomes thickened and is often regurgitant. There is a gradient across the aortic valve due to left ventricular outflow obstruction by hypertrophied muscle.

Symptoms include:

1. **Angina** – even with normal coronary arteries probably due to the increased muscle mass.

2. **Dyspnoea** – due to poor left ventricular compliance or associated mitral regurgitation.

3. **Palpitations** – atrial fibrillation and ventricular arrhythmias. There is association with Wolff–Parkinson–White syndrome and mitral valve prolapse.

4. **Syncope** – due to arrhythmias and left ventricular outflow tract obstruction.

5. **Congestive heart failure**.

6. **Systemic embolism**, which is more common if atrial fibrillation is present.

There is a risk of endocarditis and a rare familial association with atrial myxoma.

The pulse is clinically steep rising and 'jerky'. The cardiac apex may be displaced due to hypertrophy. There may be a late systolic aortic ejection murmur and a mitral regurgitant murmur.

The prognosis is worse for young persons with this condition. Annual mortality in those under 14 years of age is 6% and is 3% in the 15–45 years age group. Surgery is reserved for those with severe symptoms despite medical treatment. A myotomy is undertaken through the aortic valve to reduce the gradient. Surgery carries an operative mortality of 10–25% and death usually is due to postoperative ventricular arrhythmias. Dual-chamber pacing relieves symptoms of fatigue and breathlessness. Some patients benefit from implantable defibrillators.

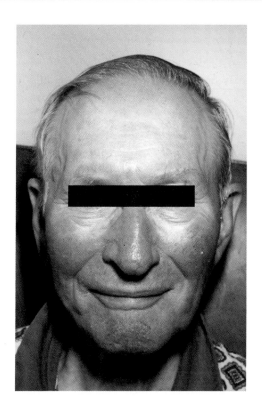

Questions

This man had a 10-year history of atrial fibrillation.

a. What is the clinical sign?
b. What is the most likely cause?
c. List two other causes.

Answers

a. A grey/violet facial pigmentation.

b. Amiodarone, is the most likely cause, especially after long-term use as in this case.

c. Other drugs that may cause skin pigmentation include: minocycline (occurs in 50% of cases after prolonged use), nifedipine, chlorpromazine chloroquine, busulphan. Arsenic (previously used for nerve, blood and skin diseases) can cause a diffuse hypermelanosis with multiple small spots of paler normal skin. Sarcoidosis can give a similar appearance.

Discussion

Amiodarone was initially used as a coronary vasodilator and anti-anginal agent. It is a class III anti-arrhythmic that prolongs the action potential duration. It is effective against supraventricular and ventricular tachyarrhthmias and it is probably the only anti-arrhythmic drug that is not negatively inotropic. Amiodarone has a long half-life (90 days) and therefore its action even if given intravenously may be delayed for several weeks. Loading doses are needed. Amiodarone is excreted by the lacrymal glands, skin and biliary tract.

Amiodarone has many side-effects, including:

1. Pneumonitis, which can progress to pulmonary fibrosis in 10% of cases. Pneumonitis is usually dose-related, steroid responsive and regresses when the drug is stopped.

2. Pro-arrhythmic – this is due to the prolongation of the QT interval. This predisposes to Torsades de pointes especially if there is hypokalaemia. Torsades de pointes is a dangerous form of ventricular tachycardia, which may progress to ventricular fibrillation. It may respond to i.v. magnesium sulphate.

3. Hepatitis (10%).

4. Neurological factors (proximal myopathy, peripheral neuropathy, tremor, impaired memory, insomnia). These side-effects are uncommon.

5. Hypo- or hyperthyroidism (5%). Amiodarone inhibits the peripheral conversion of T4 to T3. Clinically silent altered thyroid function tests occur in 10% of cases.

6. Corneal micro-deposits. These are asymptomatic and regress when the drug is stopped.

7. Photosensitivity (50%). Total sun block should be advised.

8. Slate-grey or bluish skin pigmentation. This occurs in 10% of those who had treatment for more than 18 months and will regress on withdrawal of the drug.

Amiodarone has some important interactions. It will increase the pro-thrombin time if the patient is on warfarin, the digoxin level is increased and it exacerbates the effects of beta-blockers and calcium-antagonists.

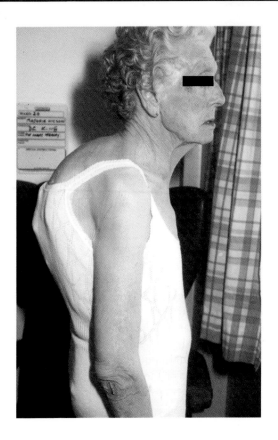

Questions

a. Describe the abnormality.
b. What is the most likely cause?
c. What is the treatment?

Answers

a. Kyphosis ('Dowager's hump') caused by wedge collapse (crush fracture) of the thoracic vertebrae.

b. Idiopathic osteoporosis.

c. Treatment should be symptomatic with analgesics such as co-proxamol. Hormone replacement therapy prevents bone loss in perimenopausal women. Cyclical etidronate (2 weeks out of 15) prevents bone loss and reduces the fracture rate. Vitamin D and calcium therapy reduces hip fracture rate in elderly people and calcitonin has been shown to decrease bone loss and fracture rate but it is expensive.

Discussion

A cause of osteoporosis should always be sought before the diagnosis of idiopathic osteoporosis is made. Causes of secondary osteoporosis include: steroids, thyrotoxicosis, Cushing's disease, multiple myeloma, hypogonadism and secondary carcinomatosis. About 30% of women and 50% of men have secondary osteoporosis. Risk factors for developing osteoporosis include smoking, obesity, reduced activity and a low calcium intake, especially in childhood. The consequences of osteoporosis, i.e. hip fractures are very costly to the NHS and also to the patient in terms of morbidity and mortality. The mortality from a hip fracture is 30% in the first 12 months.

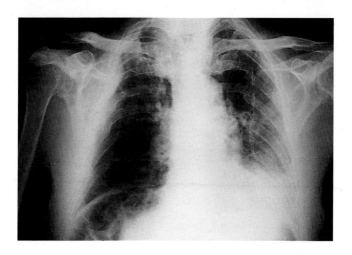

Questions

This is the chest X-ray of a 78-year-old man who had recurrent falls.

a. List three abnormalities.
b. List three causes of falls in old age.

Answers

a. Left lower lobe consolidation/collapse, fractured left ribs and Chilaiditi' sign, (bowel moves between the liver and diaphragm and decreases liver dullness. This is more common in the old and the young, and is usually asymptomatic but can cause abdominal pain).

b. Causes of falls in the elderly are multi-factorial and can be classified as follows:

1. **Accidental** (30%) – trips over furniture and carpets.

2. **Neurological** (30%), e.g. autonomic dysfunction, delayed reaction time, Parkinson's disease, stroke, epilepsy, peripheral neuropathy.

3. **Cardiovascular** (30%), e.g. postural hypotension, arrhythmias, aortic stenosis and carotid sinus syndrome.

4. **Drugs** (7%), e.g. diuretics, anti-depressants, major tranquillisers, nitrates and ACE inhibitors.

5. **Psychological** (5%), e.g. chronic brain syndrome, alcoholism and anxiety.

6. **Miscellaneous** (5%), e.g. bone disease, muscle disease, joint disease, endocrine disease and malnutrition.

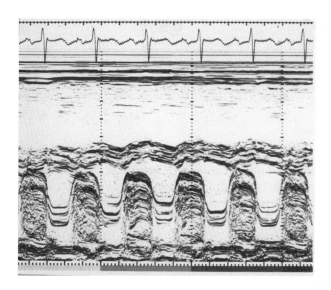

Questions

a. What is the diagnosis?
b. What is the treatment?

Answers

a. Left atrial myxoma. The mass of dense echoes between the mitral valve leaflets is the myxoma. Note the patient is in sinus rhythm.

b. Surgical removal (as soon as possible).

Discussion

A myxoma is a gelatinous, friable tumour usually attached to the septum by a pedicle. It is three times more common in the left atrium than the right. They are rarely multiple and rarely recur after removal. Left untreated, myxoma is fatal. There is a rare familial association with hypertrophic obstructive cardiomyopathy (HOCM) and lentiginosis (multiple freckles). They obstruct the mitral/tricuspid valve as they prolapse through and can cause sudden outflow obstruction. Other features include:

1. **Systemic emboli** – the tumour itself may embolise or form clot around it, which may embolise.

2. **Sudden death** – outflow obstruction or arrhythmias.

3. **Dyspnoea** – pulmonary oedema.

4. **Constitutional upset** – weight loss, myalgia, fever, raised ESR. It may mimic SABE (a diastolic murmur may be present).

5. **Arrhythmias** – atrial fibrillation may occur but is uncommon.

Although the tumour may mimic the murmur of mitral stenosis there will be no opening snap and the murmur will be variable with posture. There may be an early diastolic 'plop' sound as the tumour prolapses through the valve. The transthoracic echocardiogram usually gives the diagnosis but a transoesophageal echocardiogram is more accurate to see the exact position of the tumour and its size. Cardiac catheterisation is not necessary. Surgical removal should be arranged as soon as possible as this tumour is life threatening.

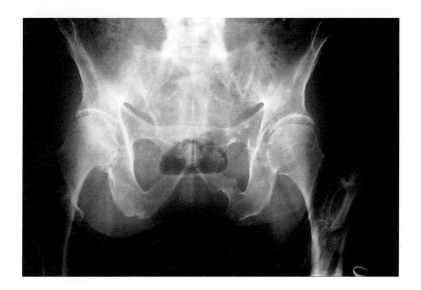

Questions

This 72-year-old man complained of diarrhoea, on and off for 6 months. He had attended his general practitioner because he developed a painful eruption on his legs.

a. What is shown on this X-ray?
b. What is the diagnosis?
c. What is the cause of his gastrointestinal symptoms?
d. What is the eruption present on his legs?
e. How should his skin lesions be treated?
f. What may be heard on auscultation of his heart?

Answers

a. There is evidence of sacroiliitis, (narrowing and irregularity of the sacroiliac joints) and there is ossification of the longitudinal ligaments of the spine, ('bamboo spine').

b. Ankylosing spondylitis.

c. Inflammatory bowel disease.

d. Erythema nodosum. Lesions are painful, erythematous macules. They can occur anywhere on the body but more commonly occur on the shins.

e. Erythema nodosum should be treated symptomatically in the first instance with non-steroidal anti-inflammatory drugs.

f. Patients with ankylosing spondylitis may have aortic regurgitation due to aortitis. The murmur of aortic regurgitation is an early diastolic murmur. If the regurgitation is severe enough, the jet of blood regurgitating onto the anterior mitral valve leaflet will produce a mid-late-diastolic mitral murmur, which is also known as an *Austin-Flint murmur.

Discussion

Ankylosing spondylitis is more common in men (8:1) and occurs in individuals between 20 and 40 years of age. There is a familial incidence and an association with *HLA-B27* (present in 96% of cases compared to 7% of the general population). It presents a peripheral asymmetrical arthritis usually involving the large weightbearing joints but the small joints of the hands and feet may also be involved. The sacroiliac joints are commonly involved, which produces backache. There is usually morning stiffness and pain is worse in the morning, which eases with exercise during the day. There is progressive spinal involvement with ultimate ossification of spinal ligaments, progressive loss of lumbar lordosis and ultimately there is a fixed kyphosis. The patient compensates for this by extension of the cervical spine in order to keep the visual axis horizontal and this produces a stooped, 'question mark' posture. The fixed spine causes a reduction in chest expansion; the patient breathes mainly by diaphragmatic movement and this causes a protuberant abdomen.

Apart from musculoskeletal features, other features of ankylosing spondylitis include:

1. **Aortic regurgitation** – this is due to aortitis and occurs in 4% of cases.

2. **Uveitis** – occurs in 30% of cases.

3. **Pulmonary fibrosis** – this is uncommon and usually occurs in the apical part of the lungs. Typically there are apical inspiratory crackles and there may be calcification and cavitation on the chest X-ray, which may lead to secondary aspergillus infection.

4. **Enteropathy** – inflammatory bowel disease, i.e. ulcerative colitis and Crohn's disease is more common in patients with ankylosing spondylitis.

5. **Psoriasis** – this is more common in people with ankylosing spondylitis than in the general population.

6. **Reiter's disease.**

7. **Cardiac conduction defects, pericarditis and cardiomyopathy** – occur in 10% of cases.

8. **Secondary amyloidosis.**

Rheumatoid factor is negative but the ESR is usually increased. *HLA-B27* is present. Typical X-ray appearances are as shown with sacroiliitis and a bamboo spine. Management includes avoiding bed rest, non-steroidal anti-inflammatory drugs, e.g. indomethacin, and posture and spinal muscle exercises to avoid deformity. Radiotherapy was previously used as it is effective in reducing pain, which is sometimes intractable, but it was associated with an increased risk of leukaemia and therefore this treatment is now not given. In severe cases, complete spinal rigidity occurs in 5 years but with appropriate multidisciplinary management 80% of cases maintain complete activity throughout their lives.

---

*Austin-Flint (1812–1886). American physician.

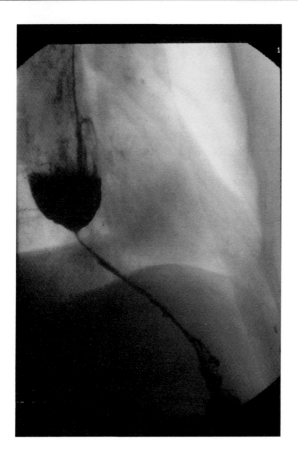

Questions

This is the barium swallow of a 70-year-old woman who had several endoscopic injections previously over a prolonged period of time.

a. What does it show?
b. What injections did she have?
c. What is the diagnosis?
d. List three symptoms she may have.

Answers

a. There is a lower tight oesophageal stricture and the oesophagus is grossly dilated proximal to this.

b. Botulinum toxin.

c. Achalasia and a benign stricture. The length of time and the injections she has had imply that the stricture is most likely benign rather than malignant. Although a benign stricture can cause a dilated oesophagus, it is most likely she has a combination of a benign stricture and achalasia. The dilatation of the oesophagus is usually not so gross with a benign stricture alone.

d. Dysphagia, chest pain and regurgitation are the most common symptoms.

Discussion

Achalasia is due to neuromuscular dysfunction of the lower end of the oesophagus with failure of relaxation and therefore progressive dilatation, tortuosity and incoordination of peristalsis of the oesophagus above this. It most commonly occurs in those over the age of 30 and it is more common in women (3:2). The symptoms are usually dysphagia, pain and regurgitation. The latter may lead to aspiration pneumonia. There is often an associated hiatus hernia and malignant change can occur in the dilated oesophagus. Treatment was previously with repeated dilatations at oesophagoscopy. A cardiomyotomy dividing the muscle of the lower end of the oesophagus and the stomach down to the mucosa also can provide satisfactory results. However, more recently the local injection of botulinum toxin has been shown to be effective. It reduces lower oesophageal sphincter tone – initially 90% of patients show an improvement and 60% show a satisfactory long-term response. Some patients receive benefit for up to 2 years. Patients over the age of 50 years have a higher response rate but repeated injections are effective. Botulinum injection is becoming more popular as oesophageal dilatation and surgery is not without risk.

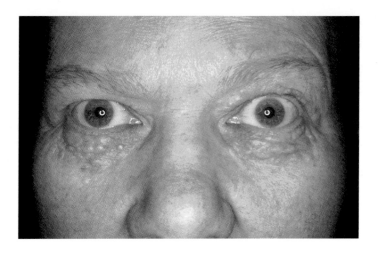

Questions

This patient complained of thirst and tiredness. She had gained weight recently and was developing alopecia. The results of investigations were as follows:

- Haemoglobin 10.6 g/dL
- MCV 104 fL
- Random blood sugar 12.4 mmol/L
- Sodium 128 mmol/L
- Potassium 3.6 mmol/L
- Urea 4.8 mmol/L.

a. What is this clinical sign?
b. What other biochemical abnormalities will be present?
c. Explain her symptoms.
d. List two other symptoms she may have.

Answers

a. Multiple xanthelasma can be seen around the eyes.

b. Hyperlipidaemia.

c. She is diabetic as she has a high random blood sugar and this can cause thirst and tiredness. Diabetes usually causes weight loss but weight gain in her case along with alopecia may be a sign of hypothyroidism, which is associated with diabetes and this may be the reason for her macrocytosis. She may also have a macrocytosis because she has pernicious anaemia, which is another association with the autoimmune diseases. Hyponatraemia may be a pseudo-hyponatraemia due to hyperlipidaemia. Both diabetes and hypothyroidism cause secondary hyperlipidaemia.

d. Angina, intermittent claudication due to peripheral vascular disease and stroke are vascular manifestations associated with hyperlipidaemia. Hyperlipidaemia can also provoke acute pancreatitis.

Discussion

Patients with hyperlipidaemia should be encouraged to adopt a low-fat diet that is high in polyunsaturated fat. They should be advised to reduce their alcohol intake and stop smoking. It is important to control any hypertension, which is often present in these patients. Oral lipid-reducing drugs may be necessary depending upon the type of hyperlipidaemia, e.g. statins, fibrates etc. It is important in particular to consider oral lipid-reducing drugs for secondary prevention where there is evidence of ischaemic heart disease as many studies have shown that their use will reduce cardiovascular morbidity and mortality.

Frederickson's classification of hyperlipoproteinaemia is as follows (types IIa, IIb and IV are the most common):

- **Type IIa** – familial hypercholesterolaemia (high cholesterol, normal triglyceride level). This type is more common in females. It may be primary or secondary to hypothyroidism, cholestatic jaundice and nephrotic syndrome. It is associated with early ischaemic heart disease: and causes corneal arcus, tendens xanthomata (Achilles) and tuborous xanthomata (on extensor surfaces).
- **Type IIb** – mixed hyperlipidaemia (increased cholesterol and increased triglyceride). Associated with ischaemic heart disease, hypothyroidism and diabetes. Causes xanthelasma and corneal arcus.

- **Type IV** – hypertriglyceridaemia (cholesterol level normal or high). This type is more common in females. It may be primary or secondary to diabetes and obesity. It is associated with gout, alcoholism and pancreatitis. It causes early ischaemic heart disease and hypertension. Eruptive cutaneous xanthomata is a feature

The following types of hyperlipoproteinaemia are rare:

- **Type I** – hyperchylomicronaemia. Causing xanthomata and pancreatitis.
- **Type II** – increased cholesterol, increased triglycerides. Causing fat deposition in palm creases.
- **Type V** – combined I and IV.

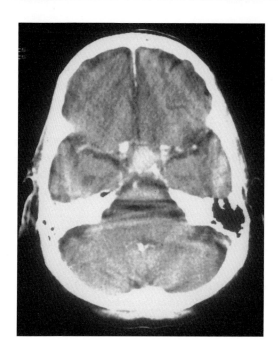

Questions

This man complained of loss of libido, weight gain and dizzy spells. On examination he looked pale, his pulse was 68 b.p.m. and regular, blood pressure 130/70 sitting and 100/60 standing. Investigations were as follows:

- Haemoglobin 11.0 g/dL
- White cell count 4.6×10^9/L
- MCV 100 fL
- Random blood sugar 3.6 mmol/L
- Sodium 127 mmol/L
- Potassium 5.8 mmol/L
- Urea 16.9 mmol/L
- TSH <0.1 mU/L.

a. What does this CT scan show?
b. What is the diagnosis?
c. List two other physical signs he may have.

Answers

a. This is a CT scan of the brain with contrast. This is known as there is a +C at the top left-hand corner of the film indicating contrast has been given. There is some artifact on the film due to movement but there is a pituitary tumour seen centrally, which is enhanced with the contrast.

b. Hypopituitarism (*Simmonds' disease). The electrolytes, i.e. low sodium, high potassium and high urea as well as the low blood sugar and postural hypotension point to hypoadrenalism. The patient also has a low thyroid-stimulating hormone (TSH) due to hypopituitarism.

c. Bitemporal hemianopia (pressure effect of the tumour on the optic chiasma), loss of body hair, pale soft skin, atrophy of genitalia and breasts.

Features of hypothyroidism include: alopecia, peri-orbital oedema, dry skin, slow relaxation of the ankle jerks. The latter is due to myotonia as a result of infiltration of the muscles by mucopolysaccharides.

Discussion

Hypopituitarism has several causes as follows:

1. Chromophobe adenoma (as in this case).
2. Iatrogenic (following hypophysectomy or eradiation).
3. Granulomatous disease (sarcoidosis, tuberculosis).
4. Secondary tumours (rare).
5. Following head injury.
6. Postpartum pituitary necrosis (†Sheehan's syndrome – rare today due to improved standards of midwifery).

The clinical picture is due to the deficiency of hormones and also pressure effects from the tumour. Deficiencies of growth hormone (GH), follicle-stimulating hormone (FSH) and luteinising hormone (LH) occur early followed by thyroid stimulating hormone (TSH) and adrenocortico-traphic hormone (ACTH). Deficiency of antidiuretic hormone (ADH) occurs latterly. Hormone deficiency causes loss of sexual function including loss of body hair and amenorrhoea. Skin pallor and depigmentation is common. Symptoms of adrenal insufficiency can occur but can be masked by those of hypothyroidism. Pressure effects include compression

*M. Simmonds (1855–1925). German physician.
†H.L. Sheehan (born 1900). Professor of pathology, Liverpool University.

of the optic chiasma and pressure on the hypothalamus can cause weight gain and fatigue.

It is important to measure all pituitary hormones, e.g. TSH, ACTH, FSH, LH and prolactin. Dynamic tests of hypothalamic pituitary function may be necessary. Treatment includes hypophysectomy if there are pressure symptoms and replacement therapy, i.e. cyclical oestrogen/progesterone in women and intramuscular depot-testosterone in men (hydrocortisone 20 mg in the morning and 20 mg at night (fludrocortisone is not required), thyroxine 100–300 mcgd.

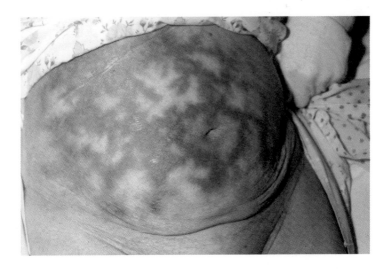

Questions

This woman had chronic abdominal pain. She had had episodes of diarrhoea on and off for 12 months. On examination of the abdomen she had a large irregular liver palpable 6 cm below the costal margin.

a. What physical sign is shown?
b. What is the cause of this?
c. What is the probable underlying diagnosis?

Answers

a. Erythema ab igne.

b. A hot water bottle to control her chronic abdominal pain has caused this appearance.

c. Her liver is most likely enlarged due to secondary metastases from an underlying colonic carcinoma, (altered bowel habit for 12 months).

Discussion

Erythema ab igne is caused by chronic infrared radiation. It occurs if the patient feels the cold more than normal and sits too close to an open fire. This is particularly common in the elderly who may be hypothyroid. The elderly feel the cold more commonly due to changes in thermoregulation with ageing and often because they live in poorer conditions and cannot afford the cost of central heating in their homes. Consequently they sit too close to an open fire. Direct heat also relieves pain and patients realise this and treat their own pain by placing hot water bottles next to their skin, which is what occurred in this case.

Erythema ab igne is similar to the pattern of livedo reticularis, which is associated with collagen vascular disease such as polyarteritis nodosa or hyperviscosity syndrome, e.g. Waldenström's macroglobulinaemia. Erythema ab igne is a pre-malignant condition and very rarely a squamous cell carcinoma can develop.

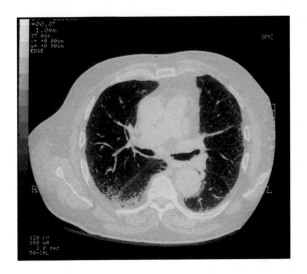

Questions

This 63-year-old man complained of increasing breathlessness. He had had a severe arthritis for many years and had retired early from his job as an electrician.

a. What does this CT scan show?
b. What is the cause in this case?
c. What chest signs may he have (list three)?
d. List three other causes of this chest condition.

Answers

a. There is evidence of fibrosis, especially posteriorly on this thoracic CT scan, more on the right side than the left. There is loss of air spaces and increased shadowing, which is a typical pattern of pulmonary fibrosis.

b. Rheumatoid disease (he has a deforming arthritis) is the most likely explanation. He may also have been exposed to asbestos in his work as an electrician, which can cause similar features but pleural plaques are usually also seen.

c. Decreased chest expansion, central cyanosis, dyspnoea, bilateral basal late fine inspiratory crackles, signs of consolidation and finger clubbing.

d. The causes of pulmonary fibrosis include:

- Cryptogenic (no indentifiable cause).
- Connective tissue disorders, e.g. rheumatoid disease, systemic lupus erythematosus, systemic sclerosis, polymyositis, dermatomyositis.
- Extrinsinc allergic alveolitis.
- Asbestosis.
- Silicosis.
- Sarcoidosis.
- Radiation fibrosis.
- Drugs, e.g. bleomycin, nitrofurantoin, amiodarone, busulphan.
- Chemicals, e.g. paraquat, beryllium and mercury.
- Ankylosing spondylitis (apical fibrosis).

Discussion

There are many associations and diseases in which pulmonary fibrosis occurs as mentioned earlier. However, when diffuse interstitial pulmonary fibrosis occurs without an apparent cause it is termed 'cryptogenic fibrosing alveolitis'. The disease usually occurs in middle-age and is more common in men. It progresses slowly but when it progresses rapidly it is known as *†Hamman–Rich syndrome.

There is clinically progressive dyspnoea and usually a dry cough without wheeze or sputum. Finger clubbing, central cyanosis, reduced chest expansion and late inspiratory crackles in the middle and lower zones are common features. Pulmonary function tests will show a restrictive pattern with a grossly reduced forced vital capacity, which gives a high or normal FEV_1:FVC ratio. The transfer factor is reduced. Chest X-ray shows diffuse bilateral basal and mid-zone reticular nodular shadowing.

The disease is progressive and steroids are usually given although the response is variable. The patient is usually hypoxic and requires constant oxygen therapy. Complications such as cor pulmonale are common. The patient usually succumbs to respiratory failure.

---

*L.V. Hamman (1877–1946). American physician.
†A.R. Rich (1893–1968). American pathologist.

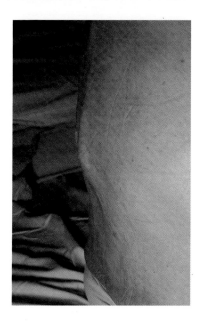

Questions

This 76-year-old woman complained of backache and rigors for 2 months. She had an area of erythema ab igne on her left hip that was excoriated where she said she had grazed herself against a wall. On examination her temperature was 38.5°C.

a. What is the physical sign?
b. What is the diagnosis?
c. Which two investigations will best confirm your diagnosis?
d. What complications may arise?

Answers

a. There is a kyphos ('gibbus') deformity of the thoracic spine due to 'wedge' collapse of the two vertebral bodies.

b. Discitis and osteomyelitis. The history indicates sepsis, the portal of entry being the skin.

c. Blood cultures and a spinal MRI scan. An MRI scan is needed to closely delineate any soft tissues in relation to the spinal cord. A plain X-ray will also confirm the diagnosis of collapse of the vertebral bodies but an MRI scan is far more helpful in locating any damage to the spinal cord and delineating a spinal abscess and tissues.

d. Spinal cord compression producing distal neurological signs is the most serious complication that can occur.

Discussion

A similar picture can occur due to tuberculosis of the spine. In these circumstances the clinical picture is of a chronic onset with lassitude, backache and weight loss but there is ultimate destruction and kyphus formation in the spinal column. X-rays will show destruction of the vertebra and intervertebral disc and may also show a paravertebral abscess shadow. The outline of psoas may be obliterated due to the abscess. Tuberculosis of the spine is also known as *Pott's disease. Similarly the infection may be due to other organisms, the commonest being *Staphylococcus*. The clinical picture is more acute with fever, rigors, malaise, nausea and vomiting. The patient is usually ill due to septicaemia. The diagnosis of staphylococcal septicaemia can be made by blood cultures but it may be possible to aspirate infective tissue under radiological control from the paravertebral area. The patient should be immobilised in a spinal brace to prevent cord compression. Intravenous antibiotics, e.g. flucloxacillin are necessary until the temperature settles and antibiotics should be given orally for a total of 6 weeks. Spinal surgery may be necessary but often is not. The spinal brace is usually required for several months until the spine is stable. If the abscess is large, drainage under X-ray control is indicated.

---

*P.Pott (1714–1788). English surgeon.

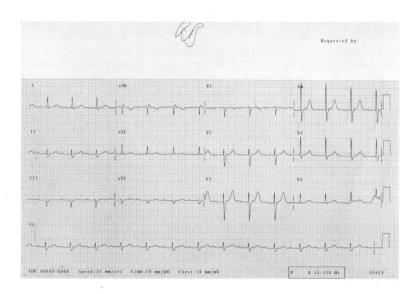

Questions

This is the ECG of a 70-year-old man who complained of recurrent blackouts.

a. What does it show?
b. What is the QRS frontal axis?
c. What is the most likely cause of his blackouts?

Answers

a. First degree heart block. The PR interval is > 0.2 s (1 cm).
b. −30°
c. Bradyarrhythmia.

He may also be having blackouts due to a tachycardia, which is ultimately reducing his cardiac output and causing cerebral hypoxia. This is a feature of the tachy–brady syndrome or sick sinus syndrome (SSS).

Discussion

Sick sinus syndrome is also referred to as sinoatrial disease and is due to impairment of sinus node activity or conduction of the impulses from the sinus node to the atria. This results in a bradycardia or sinus arrest. In some cases there is also associated tachycardias of supraventricular origin that occur as well and then it is known as the tachy-brady syndrome. The causes of sick sinus syndrome include: myocardial infarction, ischaemic heart disease, cardiomyopathy, myocarditis, drugs (e.g. digoxin) and cardiac surgery. Clinically the most common presenting symptoms are syncope, dizziness, falls and palpitations. The resting ECG may be normal or may show abnormalities as described here. A 24-hour ECG is necessary to capture an arrhythmia. If possible the patient should be given a cardio-memo so that he/she can record any arrhythmias. The probability of making the diagnosis is now increased by 8-day event recorders. Cardiac pacing is usually necessary to control symptoms except in the case of an acute myocardial infarction when sinus node function may recover after conservative management. Dual-chamber pacing increases ventricular filling and maintains an adequate cardiac output, regular atrial systole reduces the risk of thromboembolism. Long-term anti-coagulation should be considered as there is a risk of systemic embolism.

The normal QRS frontal axis is defined as −30° to +90°. The cardiac axis is the average direction of spread of the depolarisation wave through the ventricles. The causes of left axis deviation are similar to the causes of left bundle branch block, which also causes left axis deviation: ischaemic heart disease, systemic hypertension, aortic valve disease, cardiomyopathy, myocarditis. Similarly the causes of right axis deviation and right bundle branch block are the same: right ventricular strain (due to respiratory disease or chronic pulmonary emboli), atrial septal defect, myocarditis and ischaemic heart disease.

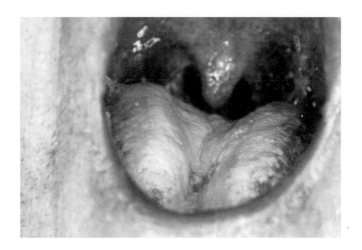

Questions

This patient complained of a sore throat.

a. What is the diagnosis?
b. List two conditions that increase susceptibility to this condition.
c. What is the treatment?

Answers

a. Oral candidiasis. White plaques are seen on the tongue, right side of the pharynx and left anterior tonsillar area.

b. Diabetes mellitus, hypoparathyroidism and conditions that suppress natural immunity, e.g. carcinoma, lymphoma, leukaemia, cytotoxic drugs, steroids and AIDS.

c. The underlying condition should be treated and oral candidiasis responds to nystatin liquid 1 ml qds.

Discussion

Candidiasis, moniliasis or thrush is a fungal infection. The areas most commonly affected are the mouth, nail folds and genitalia. The entire gastrointestinal tract may be affected and in particular oesophageal candidiasis spreads from oral candidiasis and can cause painful swallowing and dysphagia. Oesophageal candidiasis has typical radiological appearances showing an irregular ulcerated oesophagus. There is usually a reason for candidiasis, i.e. the patient has diabetes, is immunosuppressed or is generally debilitated. The diagnosis can be confirmed microbiologically by taking smears from the lesions but there is usually no need as the clinical appearance is typical.

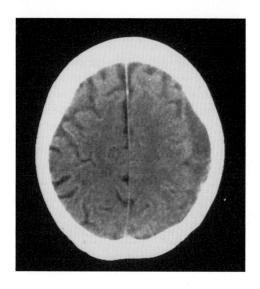

Questions

This is the CT scan of a 70-year-old woman who had recurrent headaches and episodes of confusion. She was a smoker of 20 cigarettes a day for 40 years. Other investigations were:

- Chest X-ray – enlarged left hilum
- ECG normal
- Haemoglobin 12.1 g/dL
- White cell count $4.6 \times 10^9/1$, MCV 101 fL
- ESR 100 mm/h
- ALP 300 IU/L
- AST 267 IU/L
- Gamma GT 261 IU/L
- Albumin 30 g/L
- INR 1.0
- Sodium 121 mmol/L
- Potassium 3.7 mmol/L
- Urea 16 mmol/L
- Creatinine 140 μmol/L.

a. What does the CT scan show?
b. List two possible causes of her abnormal liver function tests.
c. What other symptoms may she have (list three)?

Answers

a. There is a left subdural haematoma. The orientation of a CT scan is as if you are looking at a cross-section of the patient's head from his/her feet. On the right of the film (left side of patient) there is an area of darker colour, which is blood between the brain and the cranium. This is due to a small haematoma that is detected easily as there is clear asymmetry on the film. It is about 1 week old as fresh blood appears 'white' on CT, then becomes 'blacker'.

b. She is probably an alcoholic (macrocytosis) and has had recurrent falls producing a subdural haematoma. Another possibility for her abnormal liver function tests is liver metastases from a possible lung primary. This may also be the reason for her raised ESR and hyponatraemia.

c. 1. Drowsiness.

   2. Right-sided weakness, paraesthesia.

   3. Symptoms of raised intracranial pressure (headaches, nausea, vomiting).

   4. Symptoms related to possible bronchial carcinoma (breathlessness, haemoptysis, cerebellar syndrome, peripheral neuropathy).

   5. Symptoms related to alcoholism (falls, peripheral neuropathy).

Discussion

A subdural haematoma occurs most commonly in the elderly and in children following trauma. It may be bilateral and is due to a small venous haemorrhage. This enlarges due to the osmotic effect producing increasing absorption of the surrounding fluid. The onset is often clinically insidious and a history of previous trauma has to be carefully established with a high grade of suspicion. There is often a headache, which may be typical of raised intracranial pressure being worse in the morning. There may be intermittent confusion and the level of consciousness fluctuates. Clinical signs are usually those of raised intracranial pressure (bradycardia, hypertension and papilloedema) as well as signs due to the effect of the direct pressure of the haematoma on the brain with a contralateral weakness, e.g. hemiplegia. There is subsequent herniation of the temporal lobes through the opening of the tentorium, which gives rise to entrapment of the third cranial nerve and produces ptosis and miosis.

Treatment involves surgical removal through burr holes. Removal of the haematoma usually results in dramatic improvement in the patient.

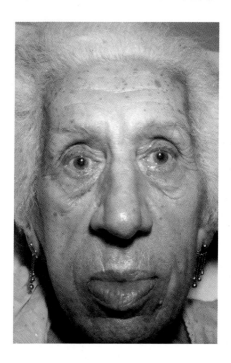

Questions

This woman complained of headaches and episodes of breathlessness on exertion. She had also awoken several times in the night with breathlessness and had developed tingling in the fingers of both hands and as a result she felt it was becoming difficult to open jam jars etc. She had seen her GP, who told her she must stop driving her car. Results of investigations were as follows:

- Chest X-ray – cardiomegaly
- ECG – left ventricular hypertrophy
- Full blood count – normal
- Random blood sugar – 12.4 mmol/L.

a. What is the diagnosis?
b. What is the cause of her breathlessness?
c. Why was she having difficulty with the activities of daily living?
d. Why did her GP tell her she must stop driving?

Answers

a. Acromegaly. There is obvious enlargement of her nose, lips, mandible and frontal bones.

b. Left ventricular failure (orthopnoea is described, which is a classical symptom of left ventricular failure). This is possibly secondary to hypertensive heart disease, which occurs in 20% of cases of acromegaly. She has evidence of longstanding hypertension with cardiomegaly on the chest X-ray and left ventricular hypertrophy on her ECG. She may also have an associated cardiomyopathy, which can occur in acromegaly and give rise to left ventricular failure.

c. She has bilateral carpal tunnel syndrome. She has weakness of her hand muscles because of this and it is the reason she is having difficulty opening jam jars etc.

d. She has a bi-temporal hemianopia, which means she is not legally permitted to drive. It is important that doctors know how to advise patients about driving under certain medical circumstances. The following publication is very useful and can be obtained from the Drivers Medical Unit, DVLA, Swansea: *For medical practitioners: At a glance guide to the current medical standards of fitness to drive* (March 1998).

Discussion

Acromegaly is caused by excessive secretion of growth hormone by an adenoma of the anterior pituitary gland. The mean age at presentation is 40 years. Growth hormone causes overgrowth of soft tissues, e.g. skin, tongue, viscera and bones and has an anti-insulin action. The patient complains of excessive sweating, acne, greasy skin, and an increase in shoe, glove and hat size. Carpal tunnel syndrome and arthralgia are common. Pressure effects cause headache, and visual field and acuity disturbance. Decreased libido, galactorrhoea, diabetes mellitus, diabetes insipidus and hypercalcaemia can also occur.

Investigations reveal a high level of circulating growth hormone not suppressed by glucose in a standard glucose tolerance test. A skull X-ray may show enlargement of the sella, large supra-orbital ridges and a protruding lower jaw. A CT scan of the head reveals a tumour and would demonstrate suprasella extension. However, MRI scanning is the investigation of choice today in cases of pituitary tumour as it is more sensitive than methods used previously. X-rays of the hands and feet show tufting of the terminal phalanges. A chest X-ray and ECG may show evidence of left ventricular hypertrophy as in this case.

Life expectancy is reduced owing to the cardiovascular complications, i.e. heart failure and arrhythmias. Trans-sphenoidal hypophysectomy is the treatment of choice but craniotomy is sometimes needed if there is suprasella extension of the tumour. Yttrium implants and external irradiation are alternatives to surgery. Bromocriptine, which reduces growth hormone and prolactin levels, may be used as an adjunct or as sole therapy in those not fit for other treatments.

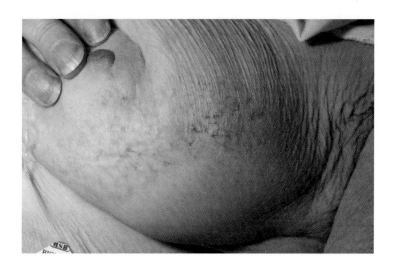

Questions

a. What is this skin lesion?
b. What other physical sign may she have?

Answers

a. Radiation dermatitis. There is also skin tethering in the sub-mammary area (left of the picture).

b. Fine inspiratory crackles in the left lung (unilateral sign) due to radiation fibrosis in the left lung. She may also have signs of recurrence of her breast tumour; breast lump, axillary/supraclavicular lymphadenopathy, hepatomegaly etc.

Discussion

Radiation dermatitis due to high-dose radiotherapy is typically a pigmented area with atrophy and telangiectasia of the skin. The condition is pre-malignant. When the dosage of radiotherapy has been sufficient to cause radiation dermatitis there is often damage of underlying tissues causing fibrosis, in this case, pulmonary fibrosis due to radiation. The clinical features are similar to other causes of pulmonary fibrosis, i.e. fine inspiratory crackles but the signs are unilateral and the chest X-ray shows a demarcated area of pulmonary fibrosis due to radiation therapy. In the case of radiation dermatitis the skin is dry and this may lead to irritation. Moisturising creams provide relief from itching etc.

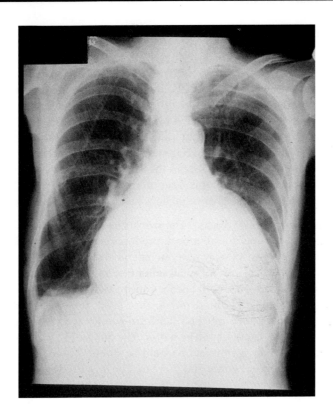

Questions

This is the chest X-ray of a 72-year-old woman who complained of dysphagia.

a. List two abnormalities on the X-ray.
b. What probable physical signs will she have? (list three).
c. What is the cause of her dysphagia?

Answers

a. There is gross cardiomegaly. There is a large left atrium and the enlarged atrial appendage is giving the left heart border a convex instead of its usual concave appearance. Of course the loss of the left heart border concavity can be due to an enlarged pulmonary artery or enlargement of the left main bronchus due to a mass. Radiological signs of an enlarged left atrium include: a straight left heart border, a double heart border on the right due to the border of the left atrium as well as the right ventricle, and the left main bronchus is elevated by the large left atrium. On this X-ray there are also *Kerley B lines at the right base, which are horizontal lines due to inter-alveolar oedema.

b. Signs of mitral valve disease. The size of the left atrium indicates that she most likely has mitral stenosis predominating over mitral regurgitation. The signs she may have include: malar flush (this is a sign of pulmonary hypertension), small volume pulse, tapping apex beat that is displaced, left parasternal heave (due to right ventricular hypertrophy), loud first heart sound and opening snap (these denote a pliable valve), mild-diastolic murmur, and pre-systolic accentuation due to increased flow caused by atrial systole. She may be in atrial fibrillation when pre-systolic accentuation would be absent. There will be a loud pulmonary second sound and there may be an early diastolic murmur of pulmonary regurgitation if there is severe pulmonary hypertension, but these are rare. She may also have a pansystolic murmur of mitral regurgitation.

c. Enlarged left atrium causing extrinsic pressure on the oesophagus.

Discussion

Mitral stenosis is always secondary to rheumatic fever although only 50% of the patients have a positive history of rheumatic fever. It is four times as common as mitral regurgitation and twice as common as mixed mitral valve disease caused by rheumatic fever. 70% of patients are female and the valve lesion may occur 2–20 years after the episode of acute rheumatic fever. In rheumatic fever the group A streptococci have antigens that cross-react with the tissue in the heart valves. Small nodules develop, the cusps thicken and stenosis occurs. Typical symptoms include: dyspnoea on exertion, orthopnoea, paroxysmal nocturnal dyspnoea, fatigue and haemoptysis due to bronchial vein rupture. Systemic embolism occurs in 30% of cases when the patient presents

*P.J. Kerley (1900–1978). British neurologist.

with atrial fibrillation. Other possible symptoms include palpitations, chest pain, dysphagia due to pressure of the left atrium on the oesophagus; and hoarseness due to pressure of the left atrium on the laryngeal nerve. Infective endocarditis is also a risk, rare in pure mitral stenosis but more common in mitral regurgitation.

Causes of mitral regurgitation include: rheumatic fever, papillary muscle dysfunction due to ischaemia, floppy mitral valve prolapse, bacterial endocarditis, cardiomyopathy, and congenital factors (e.g. those associated with a primary atrial septal defect and congenital malformations, e.g. Marfan's syndrome). The symptoms of mitral regurgitation are similar to mitral stenosis although dyspnoea is more common as is right heart failure. Mitral regurgitation predisposes to subacute bacterial endocarditis, which is more a risk than in pure mitral stenosis.

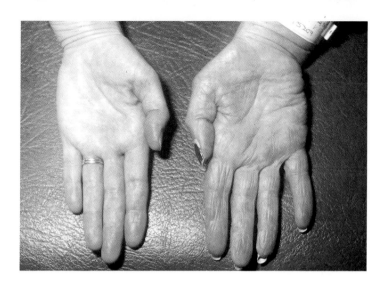

Questions

The photograph shows the hands of two separate people. The hand on the left is normal and the woman whose hand is on the right complains of a cough and she has a right ptosis.

a. What abnormality is present?
b. What is the cause of this?
c. List two other eye signs she will have.

Answers

a. There is wasting of the small muscles of the hand particularly the thenar eminence.

b. Right *Pancoast's tumour.

c. She has a right †Horners' syndrome: miosis, enophthalmos, anhydrosis and ptosis.

Discussion

The small muscles of the hand are innervated by the T1 nerve root. Causes of bilateral wasting of the small muscles of the hands are as follows:

- Atrophy due to ageing
- Syringomyelia
- Motor neurone disease
- Bilateral cervical ribs
- Rheumatoid arthritis
- Bilateral median and ulnar nerve lesions.

Causes of unilateral muscle wasting including:

- Brachial plexus trauma
- Pancoast's tumour.

A Pancoast's tumour is an apical bronchial carcinoma that is usually squamous cell. These signs (as in this case) are caused by pressure and damage to the sympathetic chain in the cervical and thoracic regions and in the T1 nerve root. Other causes of Horner syndrome include:

- Local neoplasms in the neck
- Brainstem vascular disease, e.g. lateral medullary syndrome
- Demyelinating disease
- Syringomyelia
- Carotid aneurysm
- Neck trauma.

---

*H.K. Pancoast (1875–1939). American radiologist.
†J.F. Horner (1831–1886). Swiss ophthalmologist.

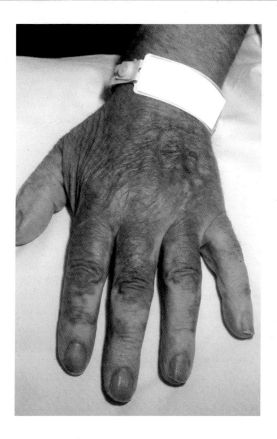

Questions

This man complained of tiredness and difficulty walking. On examination he had increased tone in his legs, weakness and hyper-reflexia. Investigations were as follows:

- Haemoglobin 8.3 g/dL
- MCV 104 fL
- White cell count 3.4×10^9/L
- Platelets 100×10^9/L
- Electrolytes normal
- ESR 4 mm/h.

a. What physical sign is shown?
b. What is the cause in this case?
c. List two other physical signs he may have in his legs.

Answers

a. Vitiligo

b. Pernicious anaemia.

c. Posterior column loss, i.e. loss of position and vibration sense, and positive *Rombergism. Reflexes may be increased in association with pyramidal signs and there is weakness. There may be a peripheral neuropathy producing absent jerks and decreased sensation to touch and tenderness on deep palpation of the calves.

Discussion

Vitiligo is the term given to areas of depigmentation of the skin. This may occur anywhere on the body and is often asymmetrical. It may occur in sites subject to friction, which are often affected by the Koebner phenomenon. Alopecia areata and premature greying of the hair are also associated with vitiligo and these signs are part of an auto immune phenomenon and therefore related to and occur in association with other autoimmune diseases, e.g. diabetes mellitus, pernicious anaemia, rheumatoid arthritis, hypothyroidism, Graves' disease, Addison's disease, systemic sclerosis, dermatomyositis, coeliac disease.

The cause of vitiligo in this case with the clinical picture and the investigations showing a macrocytic anaemia, is most likely pernicious anaemia. As well as a macrocytosis, pernicious anaemia is associated with a suppressed white cell and platelet count. The patient will have antibodies to gastric parietal cells and intrinsic factor. The neurological consequences of B_{12} deficiency are: sub-acute combined degeneration of the cord (both pyramidal tract and posterior column signs), peripheral neuropathy and rarely dementia and optic atrophy. Following the diagnosis the treatment is with B_{12} injections 1 mg daily for 1 week then 3 monthly for life. The neurological symptoms and signs improve slowly and the sensory abnormalities are more likely to resolve completely compared to the motor abnormalities, which show a more delayed and incomplete recovery.

---

*M.H. Romberg (1795–1873). German neurologist.

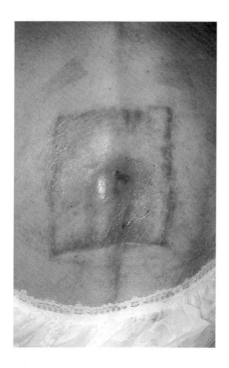

Questions

This 78-year-old woman was admitted very ill with bronchopneumonia.

a. What two events have occurred to cause this appearance?
b. What is the treatment?

Answers

a. There is a pressure sore on her kyphotic thoracic spine. She has become immobilised due to bronchopneumonia. She probably has a kyphosis secondary to osteoporosis and vertebral collapse: the kyphotic area is prone to pressure sores. There is also a well-demarcated square area over the pressure sore, which is most likely the outline of a dressing that she is allergic to. This is contact dermatitis.

b. She should be nursed as much as possible on her side, turned every hour and not allowed to put pressure on her thoracic spine. She should be nursed on a pressure-relieving mattress and the pressure area should be covered with a dressing to which she is not allergic, e.g. Granuflex.

Discussion

The prevalence of pressure sores is 4–10% in hospitalised patients. Risk is related to: old age, immobility, malnutrition, arterial disease and sensory impairment. Many risk factor assessment scales have been developed to determine how 'at-risk' some people are, e.g. the Waterlow score.

Pressure sores can be classified simply as follows:

- **Grade I** – Skin intact
- **Grade II** – Skin loss, epidermis/dermis involved
- **Grade III** – Full thickness loss and damage to subcutaneous tissues
- **Grade IV** – Extensive destruction, tissue necrosis or damage to underlying muscle or bone.

Management consists of prevention with special pressure-relieving mattresses. In patients who have already developed sores, it is important to improve health and nutrition, clean the wound with simple cleaning solutions and use simple dressings. Any infection should be treated with systemic antibiotics. Pressure sores have a significant effect on morbidity and mortality. They are under-reported and cost the NHS approximately £2 million per year.

Data
interpretation

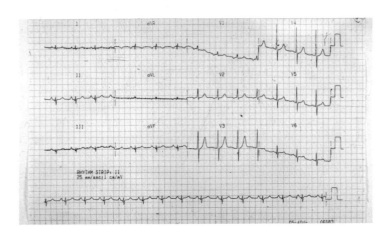

Questions

This is the ECG of a 56-year-old woman who complained of severe central chest pain 2 days previously. Her chest X-ray was normal.

a. What is the diagnosis based on this ECG?
b. How should she be managed?

Answers

a. True posterior myocardial infarction.

b. It is too late for thrombolysis, which should be given in the first 12 hours of the infarct. Risk factors should be excluded: smoking, high cholesterol levels, diabetes mellitus and hypertension. She should be given aspirin and beta-blockade should be considered if there are no contraindications. She should have an exercise stress test to determine prognosis and the need for further intervention (coronary angiography). She should also have an echocardiogram to determine systolic function. Treatment of systolic dysfunction post-myocardial infarction with ACE inhibitors has been shown to improve outcome in terms of morbidity and mortality in several trials.

Discussion

The history and findings of tall R-waves in V1 and V2 infer a true posterior myocardial infarction. The tall R-waves in V1 and V2 are the reciprocal of the Q-waves, which should be found in a lead overlying the posterior of the heart. There is no evidence of acute ischaemia on this ECG. The infarct is 2 days old.

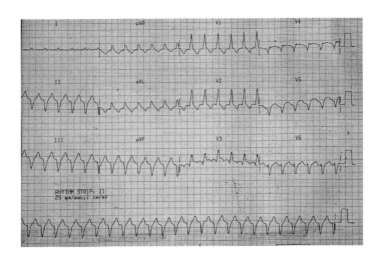

Questions

This is the ECG of a 32-year-old woman who complained of palpitations. She had had a 'flu like' illness 1 week previously.

a. What is the diagnosis?
b. What is the underlying cause in this case?
c. What is the QRS frontal axis to the nearest 15°?
d. List three other causes of the ECG diagnosis.

Answers

a. Ventricular tachycardia (VT).
b. Myocarditis.
c. Minus 75°.
d. Myocardial infarction or ischaemia

- Cardiomyopathies
- Valvular heart disease
- Mitral valve prolapse
- Drug toxicity, e.g. digoxin, quinidine
- Cardiac surgery
- Inherited conditions, e.g. Romano–Ward syndrome, Lange–Neilson syndrome
- Idiopathic.

Discussion

The most likely cause of VT in this young woman is viral as she had a 'flu like' illness and the most common virus implicated is coxsackie B. The condition is self-limiting and treated symptomatically.

Ventricular tachycardia is defined as three or more ventricular ectopic beats in rapid succession (rate 120–250 b.p.m.). The arrhythmia may be well tolerated if the patient is otherwise healthy as in this case with no underlying heart disease. It can cause shock, circulatory failure or progress to ventricular fibrillation. The ECG complex is broadened (> 0.12 s), the rate regular and there may be independent P-waves, capture or fusion beats. The differential diagnosis is supraventricular tachycardia (SVT) with bundle branch block (BBB). This does not have independent P-waves, capture or fusion beats. Capture beats occur when the atrial impulse reaches the AV node and activates the ventricles before the next discharge from the ventricular focus. This results in a narrower complex with a subsequent pause. A fusion beat occurs when the atrial impulse activates the ventricles slightly later in the cardiac cycle with simultaneous activation of the ventricular focus, giving an altered morphological complex and no pause. The RSr pattern (dominant R) in V1 favours VT as in SVT with right BBB; the pattern is rSR. In addition, the S-wave depth in V6 exceeds the R-wave and favours VT as in SVT with RBBB; the R-wave is greater than the S-wave. With the advent of adenosine this diagnostic dilemma has been aided because intravenous adenosine will convert SVT to sinus rhythm but not VT because it acts at the AV node. Adenosine has a short half-life (5–10 s) and has no lasting unwanted effects.

If VT causes shock or cardiac arrest or is drug resistant, immediate cardioversion is necessary. The first drug of choice is i.v. lignocaine. Second-line drugs include: disopyramide, flecainide and amiodarone. Only amiodarone is not negatively inotropic but its long half-life means it is not immediately effective. If drugs are ineffective and the arrhythmia is recurrent, overdrive pacing is helpful. Surgery is indicated if other methods fail when the focus is excised but this is not without risk.

There are two congenital syndromes that cause a prolongation of the QT interval and a propensity to VT: Romano–Ward syndrome (autosomal dominant) and the Lange–Neilson syndrome (autosomal recessive and associated with nerve deafness). The cause is thought to be an imbalance between left and right sympathetic innovation of the heart. Beta-blockade is often effective and left cervical sympathectomy may help prevent VT.

Questions

A 66-year-old man complained of weight loss, polyuria and left shoulder pain. His blood results were as follows:

- Haemoglobin 11.6 g/dL
- ESR 78 mm/h
- Blood glucose 8.1 mmol/L
- Albumin 23 g/L
- Calcium 2.9 mmol/L
- Urea 31.6 mmol/L
- Sodium 153 mmol/L.

a. What is his corrected calcium?
b. What is the most likely diagnosis?
c. What other investigations would you request? (name two)
d. What immediate treatment would you give?

Answers

a. Corrected calcium = 3.24 mmol/L (40–23) × 0.02 + 2.9 = 3.24 mmol/L

b. Left apical bronchial carcinoma (*Pancoast's tumour). This is the cause of the weight loss and left shoulder pain. Hypercalcaemia may be due to the secretion of a PTH-like substance from the tumour or bony secondaries.

   There may be wasting of small muscles of the left hand due to pressure on C8/T1 by the tumour. Finger clubbing may be present and symptoms of left †Horner's syndrome (ptosis, miosis, anhydrosis, enophthalmos).

c. Chest X-ray, CT scan and fine needle aspiration, and bronchoscopy.

d. Immediate treatment should be directed at correcting the calcium level. The calcium can be reduced by rehydration with i.v. 5% dextrose solution. About 6 litres should be given in the first 24 h with frusemide if necessary. Steroids reduce the calcium level in hypercalcaemia if it is secondary to malignant disease. Intravenous biphosphonates, e.g. disodium pamidronate, are very effective in lowering calcium in malignancy acting by reducing the rate of bone turnover (this action may need to be repeated). Calcitonin (IM or SC) can be used but the injections are painful and side-effects are common (flushing, nausea, vomiting, reaction at the injection site) and it is expensive.

Causes of hypercalcaemia

- Excess PTH (primary and tertiary hyperparathyroidism ectopic production by tumour)
- Excess vitamin D (self-administered)
- Sarcoidosis (increased sensitivity to vitamin D)
- Myelomatosis
- Malignancy
- Thyroid disease (hypo- or hyperthyroidism)
- Addison's disease
- Immobilised Paget's disease
- Milk-alkali syndrome.

---

*H.K. Pancoast (1875–1939). American radiologist.
†J.F.Horner (1831–1886). Swiss ophthalmologist.

Questions

A 60-year-old obese woman with diabetes and hypothyroidism complained of diarrhoea. She was taking thyroxine 50 mcg daily, gliclazide 160 mg daily and metformin 500 mg t.d.s. had recently been commenced. Her blood results were as follows:

- Sodium 98 mmol/L
- Potassium 3.1 mmol/L
- Bicarbonate 20 mmol/L
- Random blood sugar 18 mmol/L
- Urea 4.0 mmol/L.

a. What is the reason for these blood results?
b. What is the cause of her diarrhoea?

Answers

a. Pseudo-hyponatraemia, which is due to hyperlipidaemia associated with diabetes mellitus and hypothyroidism. A true sodium of this level would cause the patient to be very ill (drowsy, convulsions). Sodium ions are distributed in the aqueous phase of plasma and if there is severe hyperlipidaemia or hyperproteinaemia then the volume of distribution of the sodium ions is lower than the volume of the sample. The result is expressed taking the total volume into account. Ether extraction of the lipid would give the true sodium level.

b. The most likely cause of her diarrhoea is the recent introduction of metformin, which may also cause lactic acidosis (more common with phenformin), anorexia, nausea, vomiting and decreased B_{12} absorption. Diarrhoea can occur in diabetes due to malabsorption and autonomic neuropathy. Diarrhoea is a feature of thyrotoxicosis but it is unlikely this woman was thyrotoxic as she is only on a small dose of thyroxine and is obese, although thyroid function tests should be requested.

In the first instance metformin should be discontinued and she should see a dietician. If the diarrhoea is persistent further investigation (sigmoidoscopy and barium enema) may be necessary.

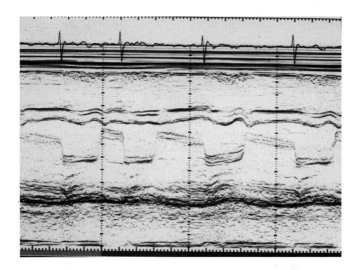

Questions

This patient presented with a transient ischaemic attack. There was no past medical history of note.

a. What is this investigation?
b. What is the diagnosis?
c. What is the treatment?

Answers

a. M-mode echocardiogram (this is a time motion recording of a beam projected through the mitral valve leaflets).

b. Mitral stenosis. The patient is in atrial fibrillation. The mitral valve leaflets are thickened and calcified. The anterior mitral valve leaflets (upper trace) has lost its classic M shape and the posterior mitral valve leaflet moves anteriorly in diastole instead of posteriorly thereby losing its mirror image (of anterior mitral valve leaflet) W shape. The total diastolic leaflet separation is reduced as fusion of the commisseures restricts opening of the leaflets. There is also evidence of aortic regurgitation seen as a 'quivering' effect on the anterior mitral valve leaflet as the regurgitant jet of blood falls onto it. This produces the *Austin Flint murmur, which is in this case clinically indistinguishable from the murmur of mitral stenosis.

c. Digoxin and lifelong warfarin.

Discussion

Surgical intervention is indicated in mitral stenosis if the mitral valve area is less than or equal to 1 cm^2 and/or the patient is symptomatic. All patients should be considered for percutaneous balloon mitral valvuloplasty. If there is evidence of a left atrial thrombus or there is valve calcification or significant mitral regurgitation then this procedure is contraindicated. The patient should be evaluated for this by transoesophageal echocardiography. If necessary the next step would be a mitral valve replacement. Studies have shown no difference in outcome when comparing balloon valvuloplasty and mitral valve surgery.

---

*Austin Flint (1812–1886) American physician.

Questions

A 23-year-old woman experienced sudden onset of headache and developed a right-sided ptosis.

a. What other signs may be present?
b. What other symptom may she have?
c. What is the diagnosis?
d. What is the most likely cause?
e. Name one investigation you would request.

Answers

a. Dilated (mydriatic) pupil that is unreactive, a divergent strabismus with the eye in the down and out position

b. Diplopia

c. Third (oculomotor) cranial nerve palsy (may be partial or complete).

d. Posterior communicating artery aneurysm (unruptured – usually painful).

e. CT scan head proceeding to cerebral arteriography before surgical clipping. Recovery of the lesion is never complete.

Discussion

The most common cause of a third cranial nerve palsy is a posterior communicating artery aneurysm. Other causes are:

1. Mononeuritis multiplex (diabetes mellitus, sarcoidosis, amyloidosis, carcinomatosis, SLE, Wegener's granulomatosis, polyarteritis nodosa)
2. Mid-brain lesions (vascular, demyelinating)
3. Syphilis
4. Carcinoma of skull base
5. Ophthalmoplegic migraine
6. Encephalitis.

Questions

A 30-year-old woman complained of recurrent falls and she was unable to comb her hair. She had had recurrent urinary tract infections. Her blood tests were as follows;

- Sodium 140 mmol/L
- Potassium 2.8 mmol/L
- Bicarbonate 15 mmol/L
- Urea 7.6 mmol/L
- Calcium 2.3 mmol/L
- Albumin 38 g/L
- Alkaline phosphatase 400 IU/L.

a. What is the reason for her symptoms?
b. What is the diagnosis?
c. Name two other symptoms she may have.
d. Name an X-ray abnormality.

Answers

a. Proximal myopathy due to osteomalacia.

b. Renal tubular acidosis.

c. Bone pain, pain from pathological fracture, renal stones due to hypercalcaemia.

d. Pathological fracture, pseudo fracture (*Milkman fracture, †Looser's zones – best seen in pubic rami), nephrocalcinosis on plain abdominal X-ray.

Discussion

There is a hypokalaemic acidosis. Hypokalaemia is usually associated with alkalosis, e.g. diuretics, vomiting (pyloric stenosis). Renal tubular acidosis is divided into two types depending on where the defect is in the proximal or distal tubule:

Type I renal tubular acidosis

Distal tubule exchanges sodium ions for potassium ions instead of hydrogen ions. The urine is alkaline and hypokalaemia is common. Nephrocalcinosis, urinary tract infections, renal stones and osteomalacia can occur. It is treated with potassium and alkalis.

Causes include:

- Congenital (autosomal dominant)
- Obstructive uropathy
- Pyelonephritis
- Hypercalcaemia.

Type II renal tubular acidosis

Proximal tubule is unable to excrete hydrogen irons. It is more common in children. Treatment with alkalis is disappointing.

Causes include:

- Wilson's disease
- Hyperparathyroidism
- Degraded tetracyclines
- Cystinosis
- ‡Fanconi's syndrome (renal rickets, glycosuria, amino acid urea and hyperphosphaturia).

Causes of hypokalaemic acidosis include:

- Renal tubular acidosis
- Diabetic coma
- Transplantation of ureters into the colon
- Severe diarrhoea
- Acetazolamide
- Forced alkaline diuresis for salicylate overdose.

---

*L.A. Milkman (1895–1951). American radiologist.
†E. Looser (1877–1936). Swiss surgeon.
‡G. Fanconi (1882–1979). Swiss paediatrician.

Questions

A 21-year-old young woman complained of sudden onset of right-sided pleuritic chest pain and breathlessness. Her arterial blood gases were:

- pH 7.35
- Pco_2 4.0 kPa
- Po_2 8.6 kPa.

a. What do the blood gases show?
b. What is the most likely cause?
c. Name one possible abnormality on her ECG.

Answers

a. Type I respiratory failure (low Pco_2 and low Po_2).

b. Pulmonary embolism (could be pneumonia but sudden onset and history favours pulmonary embolism).

c. Right bundle branch block, S1 Q3 T3, atrial fibrillation (most common arrhythmia). Sinus tachycardia is common.

Discussion

Pulmonary embolism in this young woman may have been related to the oral contraceptive pill. Other causes include:

- Previous surgery or trauma
- Prolonged bed rest
- Congestive heart failure
- Myocardial infarction
- Stroke
- Pregnancy
- Polycythaemia and thrombotic disorders.

The chest X-ray may be normal or show segmental oligaemia, linear collapse, small (usually unilateral) pleural effusion (exudate, protein level > 30 g/dl). A ventilation/perfusion scan (V/Q scan) helps with the diagnosis where there is ventilation/perfusion mismatch. However, if the lungs are abnormal to start off with due to chronic lung disease, then this makes the interpretation harder. If it is entirely normal it is useful in the exclusion of a pulmonary embolus. Pulmonary arteriography is the most precise. Spiral CT scanning has also been shown to be effective in demonstrating emboli in the pulmonary circulation. Any underlying cause of the pulmonary embolus should be removed if possible (e.g. the oral contraceptive pill) and the patient should receive anti-coagulation with warfarin for 6 months. In some cases it is prudent to continue life-long warfarin or for as long as the benefits outweigh the risks (e.g. if the patient has chronic atrial fibrillation).

Questions

A 60-year-old man complained of weakness and stiffness in his legs. He had an emergency abdominal operation 30 years previously but he could not remember what it was for. His blood tests were as follows:

- Haemoglobin 6.9 g/dL
- Bilirubin 100 μmol/L
- White cell count 2.6×10^9/L
- Platelets 128×10^9/L.

a. What is the cause of his symptoms?
b. Why is his bilirubin elevated?
c. What operation did he have 30 years previously?

Answers

a. Subacute combined degeneration of the spinal cord due to B_{12} deficiency.

b. Megaloblastic disease is often associated with low-grade haemolysis causing hyperbilirubinaemia. The white cell count and platelets are often suppressed in megaloblastic anaemia.

c. Partial gastrectomy (rendering him deficient in intrinsic factor, which is necessary for B_{12} absorption) for a perforated duodenal ulcer. The blood picture may be diamorphic as these patients are also at risk of iron deficiency anaemia.

Discussion

Neurological consequences of B_{12} deficiency are:

1. Subacute combined degeneration of the spinal cord (pyramidal signs and posterior [dorsal] column signs)
2. Peripheral neuropathy
3. Optic atrophy
4. Dementia.

Causes of B_{12} deficiency are:

1. Pernicious anaemia (parietal cell and intrinsic factor antibodies are present). This is associated with other autoimmune disease, e.g. hypoparathyroidism, primary hypothyroidism, diabetes mellitus, rheumatoid arthritis, Addison's disease and primary ovarian failure.

2. Malabsorption, bacterial overgrowth of a small bowel, partial gastrectomy, Crohn's disease (terminal ileitis), resected terminal ileum.

Treatment is with B_{12}, 1 mg intramuscularly daily for 1 week then every 3 months for life. Recovery is not always complete. Sensory features recover more completely than motor function.

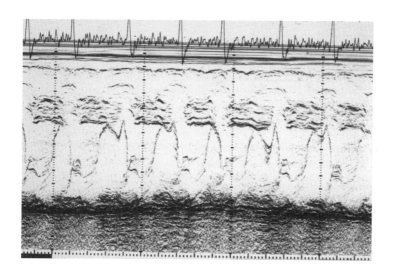

Questions

This is the M-mode echo of an asymptomatic 30-year-old woman.

a. What does it show?
b. What advice would you give?
c. What will the ausculatory findings be?

Answers

a. Mitral valve prolapse. The posterior leaflet moved backwards into the left atrium in late systole.

b. The patient is asymptomatic and she should receive endocarditis prophylaxis if there is a mitral regurgitant murmur.

c. There is a mid-systolic click due to the valve invaginating into the left atrium followed by a late systolic murmur.

Discussion

The incidence of mitral valve prolapse (floppy mitral valve) has been shown to be as high as 20% in echocardiographic studies. Postmortem studies report an incidence of 5% in females and 1% in males. It is often asymptomatic but has been associated with: atypical chest pain, paroxysmal atrial fibrillation, syncope and transient ischaemic attacks. Endocarditis is a risk if there is a murmur; this is due to the progressive stretching of the mitral valve leaflets and the chorda are also involved. The tricuspid valve may also prolapse. It is associated with other conditions: Turner's syndrome, *Marfan's syndrome, secundum ASD, Osteogenesis imperfecta, HOCM, WPW syndrome, patent ductus arteriosis.

Marfan's syndrome consists of the following features: tall stature, arm span > height, arachnodactyly, high arched palate, aortic regurgitation, coarctation of the aorta, mitral valve prolapse, propensity to dissecting aneurysms, hyperextensible joints, iridodonesis, upward lens dislocation, myopia. The syndrome is autosomal dominant.

---

*E.J.A. Marfan (1858–1942). French paediatrician.

Questions

A 58-year-old man complained of a 6-week history of increasing breathlessness and generalised joint pains. The results of investigations were:

- FEV$_1$ 1.4 litres
- VC 1.7 litres
- Transfer factor 2.8 mmol/min/kPa
- ESR 90 mm/h
- Po$_2$ 7 kPa
- Pco$_2$ 3.9 kPa.

a. What is the diagnosis?
b. What is the treatment?

Answers

a. Cryptogenic fibrosing alveolitis (*Hamman–†Rich syndrome).
b. Steroids 40 mg o.d. for 2 months then decreasing to a maintenance dose

Improvement is seen in two-thirds of cases, particularly in the young and those who suffered an acute onset, azathioprine or cyclophosphamide, oxygen, and treatment of infection and heart failure as disease progresses.

Discussion

The cause is unknown and it is more common in middle-aged individuals. There is a restrictive lung defect with hypoxia and hypocapnoea. The transfer factor is always reduced. The patient is easily dyspnoeic, cyanosed and has finger clubbing. There are inspiratory crackles (usually late inspiratory). The chest X-ray shows haziness at both bases, elevated diaphragm, generalised micronodular shadowing or a 'honeycomb' appearance. Associations include: polyarthritis (10%), chronic active hepatitis (5–10%), thyroid disease, anti-nuclear factor (30%), rheumatoid factor (50%), increased IgG levels and an increased ESR.

Causes of pulmonary fibrosis:
- Industrial lung disease
- Extrinsic allergic alveolitis
- Sarcoidosis
- Bronchiectasis
- Chronic left ventricular failure (mitral stenosis)
- Lymphangitis carcinomatosa
- Drugs (busulphan, bleomycin, amiodarone, nitrofurantoin).
- Multi-system disorders (rheumatoid arthritis, systemic sclerosis, SLE, ankylosing spondylitis, polymyositis, Sjögrens' syndrome).
- Poisons (paraquat)
- Uraemia.

---

*L.V. Hamman (1877–1946). American physician.
†A.R. Rich (1893–1968). American pathologist.

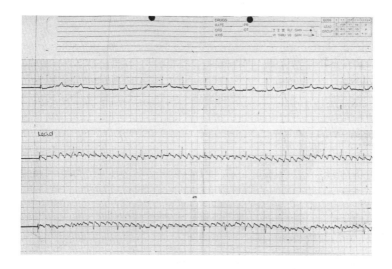

Questions

This is the ECG of a 50-year-old woman who presented with weight loss, increased appetite and anxiety.

a. What does this ECG show?
b. What is the cause in this case?
c. List three clinical signs she may have.
d. Name two other possible causes of this ECG finding.

Answers

a. Atrial flutter with variable AV block and a ventricular rate of 100 b.p.m.

b. Thyrotoxicosis.

c. Goitre (+/– bruit), eye signs (exophthalmos, lid retraction, lid lag), fine tremor, hot moist palms, proximal myopathy, pre-tibial myxoedema (1% of cases).

d. Causes of atrial flutter are the same as atrial fibrillation:

- Rheumatic heart disease
- Myocardial disease (infarction, cardiomyopathy, myocarditis, hypertension)
- Hyperthyroidism
- Sick sinus syndrome
- Atrial septal defect
- Constrictive pericarditis
- Pulmonary embolism
- Bronchial carcinoma
- Pneumonia
- Idiopathic causes.

Discussion

In atrial flutter the atrial discharge rate is about 300/min. A degree of AV block usually occurs producing F-waves, which are best seen in leads II and VI and produce a 'saw tooth' appearance. If the ventricular rate is fast the AV block can be increased by carotid sinus massage, i.v. verapamil or adenosine, which will reveal the underlying flutter waves. The rate in atrial flutter is often more difficult to control than in atrial fibrillation and the cardiac output will be compromised. Atrial flutter can almost always be terminated by low energy, syncronised DC shock (25–50 J). An alternative is rapid right atrial pacing. Anti-coagulation with heparin is advised for recent onset atrial flutter prior to cardioversion. Patients with chronic atrial flutter/fibrillation in whom cardioversion is not successful should receive digoxin as the first drug of choice to control the ventricular rate and lifelong warfarin to reduce the risk of thromboembolism. The risk of stroke in non-rheumatic atrial fibrillation is increased five times and 17 times when associated with rheumatic mitral valve disease. The risk of thrombosis is greater if the left atrial size is greater and left ventricular function is reduced.

Questions

A 70-year-old woman complained of severe pain in her feet and a swollen right knee. The results of investigations were:

- Haemoglobin 20.5 g/dL
- White cell count 18×10^9/L
- Platelets 500×10^9/L.

a. What is the cause of the pain in her feet?
b. How would you confirm the diagnosis?
c. Name two associations/complications.
d. What is the other diagnosis?

Answers

a. Gout.

b. Raised uric acid level. Aspirate from the right knee should reveal negatively birefringent crystals of monosodium urate viewed by polarised light.

c. Renal stones (uric acid stones), chronic renal failure (chronic urate nephropathy), hypertension, ischaemic heart disease, diabetes, hyperlipidaemia and obesity are more common in patients with hyperuricaemia.

d. Polycythaemia rubra vera.

Discussion

Gout can be acute or chronic and is characterised by arthritis associated with hyperuricaemia. Hyperuricaemia is however more common alone than when associated with clinical gout. The big toe is most commonly affected in the first attack followed by the tarsus and knee. More than one joint may be affected. In the acute attack the pain is sudden and there is inflammation and erythema of the joint, which is very tender. More than one joint may be affected. The arthritis is usually asymmetrical. In chronic gout, tophi may appear, especially on the cartilage of the ears and close to joints if left untreated.

Gout may be *primary* when it is due to an inborn error of purine metabolism, which most commonly affects men (6:1). It is familial in 30% of cases and may result from excessive consumption of purine-containing food. It is uncommon in pre-menopausal women. Gout may be *secondary* when there is increased purine turnover and hence an increase in serum uric acid, e.g. in myeloproliferative disease. This occurs particularly after treatment with cytotoxic drugs when the serum uric acid and urea rise as a result of tissue destruction. The patients should receive prophylaxis (allopurinol). Drugs may cause hyperuricaemia and gout, e.g. diuretics, salicylates. Chronic renal failure causes hyperuricaemia due to reduced renal excretion but is rarely associated with clinical gout.

Treatment of the acute attack includes non-steroidal anti-inflammatory drugs and if these cannot be tolerated colchicine is effective. If gout is recurrent then allopurinol should be given prophylactically. This inhibits xanthine oxidase and therefore blocks the metabolic pathway of uric acid. When allopurinol is commenced non-steroidal anti-inflammatory drugs should be given for 6 weeks to prevent acute attacks as allopurinol increases urate levels in the synovial fluid and can paradoxically produce an acute attack of gout on introduction.

Questions

A 60-year-old woman complained of weakness and tingling in her arms. On examination she had wasting of the small muscles of her hands, generalised hyper-reflexia and limited neck movements. The Cerebrospinal fluid (CSF) clotted. CSF results were as follows:

- Pressure = 17 cm H_2O
- protein = 3.8 g/L
- No cells
- Glucose = 4.8 mmol/L (blood glucose 5.5 mmol/L)
- Xanthochromia.

a. What is the most likely cause?
b. List two other possible causes of this protein level.
c. Why did the CSF clot?

Answers

a. Spinal cord obstruction (*Froin's syndrome) due to cervical spine disease.

b. Vascular lesions, tumours, hypothyroidism, diabetes. Guillain–Barré syndrome gives much higher protein levels (30–100 g/L). Viral meningitis results in lower protein levels (0.5–1 g/L) with a lymphocytosis and a low/normal sugar. Bacterial meningitis causes a high protein value (1–5 g/L) in the CSF but there are polymorphs and a very low or absent glucose concentration.

c. High fibrinogen content.

Discussions

Froin's syndrome was described in 1903 as 'high protein content in the CSF associated with xanthochromia and coagulation due to obstruction of the spinal subarachnoid space'. Upper motor neurone signs in all limbs point to a high spinal cord lesion. Wasting of the hand muscles may be due to lower motor neurone involvement and/or disuse atrophy. There may be sensory changes and ultimately a sensory level. A cervical myelogram and/or MRI scan is necessary. Surgical cervical spine fusion may be necessary to stop deterioration but this is not without risk.

---

*G. Froin (born 1874). French physician.

Questions

A 62-year-old vagrant was brought into casualty by the police after he was found unconscious. He had a fit on arrival. His results were as follows:

- Sodium 101 mmol/L
- Potassium 4.4 mmol/L
- Urea 1.3 mmol/L
- Protein 50 g/L
- Random blood sugar 6.8 mmol/L
- Chest X-ray – cystic lesion left apex.

a. Name two possible causes of the appearance on the chest X-ray.
b. Why did he have a fit?
c. What is the reason for his electrolyte disturbance?
d. How would you confirm this?
e. What is the treatment?

Answers

a. Pulmonary tuberculosis, cavitating carcinoma of lung.

b. Probably secondary to hyponatraemia. Tuberculous meningitis and brain secondaries must be considered.

c. Inappropriate antidiuretic hormone (ADH) secretion.

d. Serum osmolarity is usually < 240 mmol/L (in this case 218.4 mosm/L, 2 sodium + 2 potassium + urea + glucose) and the urine osmolarity is inappropriately higher than the serum osmolarity (350–400 mosm/L).

e. Fluid restriction and treatment of the underlying cause. Demeclocycline directly blocks the renal tubular effect of ADH given in a dose of 0.9–1.2 g daily initially in divided doses (maintenance dose 600 mg/d).

Discussion

This man's electrolytes show evidence of haemodilution (water intoxication) (low sodium, low urea, low protein). A low sodium (below 125 mmol/L) can cause confusion, drowsiness, fits and coma.

Causes of haemodilution:

1. Inappropriate ADH secretion
2. Salt depletion (diarrhoea and vomiting)
3. Water overload
4. Hypothyroidism
5. Renal failure.

Causes of inappropriate ADH secretion:

1. Ectopic ADH production
   a. Lung cancer (usually oat cell)
   b. Pulmonary tuberculosis
   c. Pancreatic carcinoma.

2. Excessive pituitary ADH
   a. Pneumonia (the most common cause of low sodium)
   b. Positive pressure ventilation
   c. Head injury
   d. Cerebral haemorrhage
   e. Meningitis/encephalitis
   f. Congestive heart failure
   g. Hypothyroidism
   h. Hodgkin's disease.

3. Drugs: chlorpropamide, tricyclic anti-depressants, thiazides, vincristine (sensitises renal tubules to ADH).

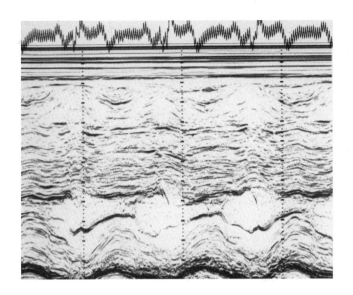

Questions

a. Name three abnormalities.
b. What is the diagnosis?

Answers

a. The intraventricular septum is hypertrophied and immobile. The posterior wall is also hypertrophied. The left ventricular cavity is small. There is systolic anterior movement (SAM) of the mitral valve apparatus. This abrupt displacement of the mitral valve to the septum and septal hypertrophy are the cause of outflow obstruction.

b. Hypertrophic obstruction cardiomyopathy (HOCM).

Discussion

(See Photographic case 20)

The ratio of septal thickness to that of the posterior wall is used as a diagnostic criteria and values equal to or more than 1.5–1 are considered diagnostic. The septal thickness should be at least 1.4 cm before the diagnosis is considered.

Questions

A 40-year-old woman attended her GP complaining of tiredness. He took some blood tests and is telephoned the next day with the results. He contacted the hospital for advice. The test results were:

- Haemoglobin 9.1 g/dL
- White cell count 7×10^9/L
- Platelets 500×10^9/L
- MCV 70 fl
- Sodium 140 mmol/L
- Potassium 8.1 mmol/L
- Urea 1.3 mmol/L
- Phosphate 1.9 mmol/L.

a. What is the likely cause of these result?
b. What is the management of this condition?

Answers

a. Iron deficiency anaemia has many causes but menorrhagia is a common cause in this age group. A cause should be sought. It is likely the blood sample was either haemolysed or left overnight to produce increased potassium and phosphate levels, which leak out of the red cells. The electrolytes should be repeated.

b. Oral ferrous sulphate and find the underlying cause.

Discussion

The elevated platelet count implies bleeding associated with iron deficiency anaemia in this case, which causes a hypochromic microcytic blood picture.

Causes of iron deficiency anaemia
1. Blood loss

   - Menorrhagia
   - Gastrointestinal loss (peptic ulcers, hiatus hernia, carcinoma of stomach, rectum, colon etc., inflammatory bowel disease).

2. Poor diet (more common in the elderly).
3. Increased demand for iron (growth, pregnancy).
4. Malabsorption (many causes and this occurs in most cases).

Questions

A 52-year-old man complained of malaise, anorexia and a sharp right-sided chest pain. His temperature was 38°C. He also had an anterior chest pain relieved by sitting upright. He had had central chest pain 8 weeks previously. His blood results were as follows:

- Haemoglobin 10.1 g/dL
- White cell count $17 \times 10^9/L$
- MCV 88 fL
- MCH 30 pg
- ESR 91 mm/h.

a. What is the cause of his current chest pain?
b. What was the cause of his pain 8 weeks previously?
c. What is the diagnosis?
d. What is the management?

Answers

a. Pleurisy and pericarditis (pericardial pain is often postural as in this case).
b. Myocardial infarction.
c. *Dressler's syndrome.
d. Non-steroidal anti-inflammatory drugs and steroids.

Discussion

Dressler's syndrome is a syndrome of pericarditis, pleurisy and fever 2–8 weeks after a myocardial infarction. It is associated with anaemia and a high ESR and tends to be recurrent. It is thought to be an autoimmune reaction to exposed myocardial antigens and affects up to 5% of infarcts. Antimyocardial antibodies are present but are not clinically useful. Treatment is symptomatic with non-steroidal anti-inflammatory drugs and steroids. Steroids may be needed for several months.

*W. Dressler (1890–1969). American physician.

Questions

A 15-year-old boy complained of colicky abdominal pain, abdominal distension and vomiting. He had a rash on his buttocks and ankles. Investigation results were as follows:

- Urine blood +++
- Protein +++
- ESR 71 mm/h
- Haemoglobin 9.8 g/dL
- MCV 74 fL
- Platelets $600 \times 10^9/1$
- Abdominal X-ray showed fluid levels.

a. What is the cause of his abdominal symptoms?
b. What kind of rash will he have?
c. Explain his results.
d. What is the diagnosis?

Answers

(a) Intestinal obstruction due to intussusception.

(b) Purpuric.

(c) ● Urine – glomerulonephritis
   ● Abdominal X-ray – intestinal obstruction
   ● ESR – inflammatory process, non-specific
   ● Full blood count – iron deficiency anaemia due to blood loss
     (increased platelets).

(d) *†Henoch–Schönlein purpura.

Discussion

Henoch–Schönlein syndrome occurs more commonly in boys aged 5–15 years. It consists of a purpuric rash (buttocks and ankles), urticaria, fever, polyarthritis (ankles, knees, hips, wrists and elbows), glomerulonephritis (renal failure is uncommon), gastrointestinal bleeds and intussusception. It is preceded by an upper respiratory tract infection in 90% of cases but beta haemolytic streptococci are only isolated in 30%. There is a widespread vasculitis. The bowel is oedematous and inflamed causing bleeding and obstruction. Treatment is symptomatic with non-steroidal anti-inflammatory drugs. Steroids are helpful for gastrointestinal symptoms. It is self-limiting and lasts 1–2 months and can recur. The prognosis is worse in adults.

---

*E. H. Henoch (1820–1910). German paediatrician.
†J. L. Schönlein (1793–1864). German physician.

Questions

A 50-year-old woman presented with melaena. She was noted to have a systolic murmur. Some months later she had cardiac catheter studies, which yielded the following results (normal range values are in parentheses):

- Right atrium 4 (0–8) mmHg
- Right ventricle 26/6 (15–30/0–8) mmHg
- Pulmonary artery 31/17 (15–30/6–16) mmHg
- Left ventricle 210/6 (90–140/4–12) mmHg
- Cardiac index 1.6 l/min/m² (2.8–4.2 l/min/m²)
- Ejection fraction 30% (60–70%)
- Blood pressure 110/70

a. What is the cardiac defect?
b. Name an abnormality on her ECG.
c. What is the management?
d. What is the likely cause of her melaena?

Answers

a. Aortic stenosis. There is a difference in the systolic blood pressure and left ventricular systolic pressure of 100 mmHg, which represents critical aortic stenosis.

b. Left ventricular strain pattern (left ventricular hypertrophy, left bundle branch block) left atrial hypertrophy.

c. Aortic valve replacement.

d. Angiodysplasia. There is an association with aortic stenosis. Other causes of gastrointestinal bleeding should certainly be considered and a gastroscopy and barium enema is required. Coeliac axis angiography during the bleed may reveal the area of angiodysplasia, which occurs more commonly in the right hemicolon.

Discussion

Aortic stenosis may be asymptomatic. Symptoms occur late and may include: angina, syncope and dyspnoea. Symptoms and a gradient of > 50 mmHg across the valve, which can be measured on Doppler echocardiography are associated with life expectancy of 18 months to 3 years without surgery. Sudden death occurs due to ventricular arrhythmias and left ventricular failure. Cardiac catheterisation is the gold standard for assessing the severity of the aortic stenosis.

Causes of aortic stenosis are rheumatic heart disease (there may be associated regurgitation and mitral valve disease), calcified congenital bicuspid valve (more common in men), calcific degeneration in the elderly. Clinically the patient has a plateau pulse, a low blood pressure and reduced pulse pressure. The apex beat may be displaced due to left ventricular hypertrophy and there may be evidence of left ventricular failure. Endocarditis prophylaxis is required.

Questions

A 68-year-old woman developed rigors and an elevated tender red facial rash on her nose and cheek. Her blood tests were as follows:

- Sodium 141 mmol/L
- Urea 20 mmol/L
- Haemoglobin 9.1 g/dL
- White cell count 15.8×10^9/L, blasts 96%, neutrophils 1%.
- Platelets 36×10^9/L.

a. What is the rash?
b. What is the other diagnosis?

Answers

a. Erysipelas.
b. Acute myeloid leukaemia.

Discussion

Erysipelas is caused by group A haemolytic streptococci. It tends to occur in patients over the age of 40 years and the face and lower limbs are the most common sites of infection. The organism is often carried in the patient's nose and enters through a break in the skin. It is therefore more common in certain conditions where there is an obvious portal of entry, e.g. varicose ulceration and eczema. Other predisposing factors as in this case include immunosuppression due to other diseases, e.g. leukaemia, lymphoma or immunosuppression due to drugs. The classical distribution of erysipelas is a 'butterfly' rash on the face. There is erythema and oedema of the skin over the nose and cheeks, which is often symmetrical. The patient is usually unwell and toxic with a high temperature due to streptococcal septicaemia. The differential diagnosis is of maxillary zoster but this rash is usually unilateral or the rash of systemic lupus erythematosus. However, in this disease the patient usually has no other signs of systemic infection.

Acute myeloid leukaemia is more common in adults and rare in children. It occurs when there is a proliferation of an abnormal blast cell in the bone marrow, which is finally replaced by blasts that result in bone marrow failure. Blast cells are the precursors of normal white cells seen in the peripheral blood. Blast cells are not seen in the peripheral blood in normal circumstances but in acute leukaemia the abnormal blast cells spill out of the marrow. The normal differential white cell count is: neutrophils 40–75%, lymphocytes 20–45%, eosinophils 1–6%, basophils < 6% and monocytes 2–10%. In this case there is a slightly elevated total white cell count but the differential count is abnormal with a high proportion of blasts. The platelet count is reduced due to marrow suppression. There may be other abnormal cells in the peripheral blood, e.g. promyelocytes, myelocytes, agranular neutrophils. The bone marrow is hypercellular with a proliferation of leukaemic blast cells, which typically amount to > 75% of the total. The clinical features of acute leukaemia can be grouped as follows:

1. Clinical features due to bone marrow failure:

   ● Infection, e.g. erysipelas as in this case, respiratory, throat or gastrointestinal infections

- Tiredness, dyspnoea malaise due to anaemia
- Abnormal bleeding due to thrombocytopenia, e.g. purpura, bruises, gastrointestinal bleeding, bleeding gums.

2. Clinical features due to organ infiltration:

- Hepatosplenomegaly
- Lymphadenopathy.

Treatment is of the consequences of the leukaemia, in this case the patient should receive i.v. penicillin after blood cultures have been taken and the diagnosis confirmed. Supportive therapy is often required, e.g. i.v. fluids. Cyclical cytotoxic drug therapy is necessary to treat the acute leukaemia and supportive transfusions may be necessary. Bone marrow transplantation should be considered for young people in the first remission.

Questions

A 27-year-old woman complained of weakness, anorexia and diarrhoea for 6 weeks. There was no significant past history of note, although her mother had a history of thyroid disease. Investigations were as follows:

- Sodium 128 mmol/L
- Potassium 5.6 mmol/L
- Urea 18.3 mmol/L
- Random blood sugar 3.9 mmol/L
- TSH 20 IU/L
- Random serum cortisol 250 nmol/L (normal range 200–700 nmol/L)
- Urine dip testing = protein ++.

a. What is the most important investigation to request next?
b. What is the diagnosis?

Answers

a. Short synacthen test or serum ACTH level.
b. Addison's disease.

Discussion

Addison's disease is hypoadrenalism due to failure of the adrenal glands. It is usually due to autoimmune adrenal destruction and is associated with other autoimmune diseases, e.g. diabetes mellitus, pernicious anaemia, thyroid disease etc. There is an association with *HLA-B8* and *HLA-DW3*. The adrenal glands may also fail due to destruction from infiltrative disorders, e.g. secondary carcinoma, leukaemia, Hodgkin's lymphoma or they may be destroyed by other diseases, e.g. tuberculosis, haemochromatosis, amyloidosis and histoplasmosis. Another rare cause of adrenal failure is bilateral adrenal haemorrhage associated with acute meningococcal septicaemia (Waterhouse–Friderichsen syndrome).

Hypoadrenalism is more common in women. The patient may present acutely with abdominal pain, fever, hypotension and collapse, which is known as an 'Addisonian crisis'. This condition is life-threatening. The onset is more often chronic and insidious with non-specific symptoms of weakness and fatigue, weight loss, nausea and abdominal pain. There is often pigmentation of the skin, especially the mucus membranes (mouth), palmar creases, nipples, genitalia and areas subject to increased pressure, e.g. elbows. The patient usually has evidence of postural hypotension and typical electrolyte abnormalities of hyponatraemia, hyperkalaemia and haemoconcentration. There is often eosinophilia and a high urine sodium level. Plasma cortisol may be normal as in this case and it is not a useful diagnostic test. The most sensitive test is a high plasma ACTH, although this takes some time and is expensive. A more available test that is cheap and sensitive is the short Synacthen test in which 250 mcg of synthetic ACTH (Synacthen) is injected intramuscularly after fasting serum cortisol is taken at 9 a.m. The serum cortisol is then measured again after 1 hour. In hypoadrenalism there is little or no rise in the levels as the failing adrenal glands cannot produce cortisol in response to ACTH. In this case the TSH is elevated and can be high in untreated hypoadrenalism. Thyroxine should not be given until the patient receives adequate treatment for hypoadrenalism.

Treatment of Addisonian crisis includes immediate i.v. saline and i.v. hydrocortisone. Treatment should begin immediately as the condition is life threatening even before the results of blood cortisol levels are available. Maintenance treatment includes hydrocortisone 20 mg in the morning and 10 mg at night (this is to mimic the diurnal variation in glucocorticoid secretion by the adrenal glands) and fludrocortisone 0.1 mg/od. During periods of stress, i.e. intercurrent infections the patient should be advised to double the dose of hydrocortisone, which is the normal physiological response to illness. There is no need to alter the dose of the fludrocortisone. If the patient is unwell and develops nausea and vomiting parenteral administration of hydrocortisone will be required.

Questions

A 22-year-old man developed testicular swelling, neck stiffness and photophobia. Investigations were as follows:

- CSF
  - Glucose 5.2 mmol/L
  - Protein 0.8 g/L
  - Lymphocytes 20
  - Polymorphs 0
- Random blood sugar 5.6 mmol/L
- Sodium 140 mmol/L
- Potassium 4.0 mmol/L
- Urea 5.0 mmol/L.

a. What is the diagnosis?
b. What is the treatment?
c. Name one complication.

Answers

a. Mumps meningitis. The CSF indicates a viral meningitis and testicular swelling points to the mumps virus.

b. Treatment is symptomatic with analgesia and i.v. fluids and if necessary treatment of secondary bacterial infection.

c. Sterility.

Discussion

The most common viruses causing meningitis are coxsackie virus and echo virus. Other viruses causing meningitis include: mumps, herpes simplex and lymphocytic chorio meningitis viruses (the last two are rare). In other parts of the world the polio and arbo viruses are important causes of meningitis.

Viral meningitis occurs mainly in young adults who present with sudden onset of fever, headache, nausea, vomiting, neck stiffness and photophobia. *Kernig's sign is usually positive – this is a sign of meningeal irritation just as neck stiffness is. The hip and knee are flexed, and extension of the knee causes pain and spasm in the hamstring muscles.

The cerebrospinal fluid protein in viral meningitis is elevated (0.5–1 g/L) but not as high as the protein level seen in bacterial meningitis (1–3 g/L). The CSF sugar is normal and the CSF white cell count usually shows a lymphocytosis. In bacterial meningitis the CSF sugar is very low and there is excess of polymorphs. The virus can be isolated from the CSF, urine or a throat swab and there is usually a rising antibody titre in paired sera. It is important to distinguish viral meningitis from tuberculous meningitis and fungal infections. Treatment is symptomatic. It is uncommon as most people have had mumps parotitis in childhood.

Normal CSF:

- Protein 0.2–0.5 g/L
- Cells < 5 lymphocytes per mm^3
- Glucose 2.2–4.4 mmol/L (or blood sugar minus 1.7). It is important to correlate the blood glucose with the CSF glucose.

---

*V.M. Kernig (1840–1917). Russian physician.

Questions

A 39-year-old woman complained of generalised arthralgia and alopecia. She had suffered Raynaud's disease for 2 years and had a history of depression. Investigations were as follows:

- Haemoglobin 10.1 g/dL
- White cell count 6.1 × 10⁹/L
- Platelets 100 × 10⁹/L
- Reticulocytes 4%
- ESR 90 mm/h
- MCV 100 fL
- Sodium 136 mmol/L
- Potassium 5.8 mmol/L
- Urea 30 mmol/L
- Creatinine 400 µmol/L
- Bilirubin 50 µmol/L
- ALP 82 IU/L
- AST 21 IU/L
- ECG – left ventricular hypertrophy.
- Chest X-ray normal

a. What is the diagnosis?
b. What complications have developed (list three)?
c. What specific investigation will confirm the diagnosis?
d. What is the treatment?

Answers

a. Systemic lupus erythematosus

b. Haemolytic anaemia, renal failure, hypertension. Haemolytic anaemia is evident from the anaemia, macrocytosis, reticulocytosis and hyperbilirubinaemia. Hypertension that is secondary to renal involvement has caused left ventricular hypertrophy on the ECG. However, this may be due to an associated cardiomyopathy.

c. Antibodies to double-stranded DNA are diagnostic.

d. Treatment is with high dose steroids and azathioprine may be used as a steroid sparing agent.

Discussion

Systemic lupus erythematosus is a connective tissue disorder and 90% of cases occur in women aged 20–40 years. The condition is exacerbated by infections and sunlight. The onset may be insidious with malaise, weight loss and general ill health. It is a multi-system disorder and the symptoms and signs can be grouped as follows:

1. **Skin** – butterfly rash is the most common feature. Photosensitivity, alopecia, telangiectasia, nail fold infarcts, Raynaud's phenomenon and non-specific erythema may occur.
2. **Joints** – Symmetrical polyarthralgia, which may mimic rheumatoid arthritis. It is uncommonly erosive and deforming.
3. **Respiratory system** – pleural effusions, consolidation, linear collapse, fibrosis, pleurisy.
4. **Renal tract** – nephrotic syndrome, nephritic syndrome. Hypertension occurs in 50% of cases.
5. **Cardiovascular system** – pericarditis, cardiomyopathy, non-bacterial endocarditis (*Libman–†Sacks endocarditis).
6. **Nervous system** – Mononeuritis multiplex, peripheral neuropathy, epilepsy, neuro-psychiatric (depression, phobias, confusion, hallucinations).
7. **Haematological system** – Autoimmune haemolytic anaemia, thrombocytopenia, leucopenia, raised ESR.
8. **Lymphatic system** – lymphadenopathy, hepatosplenomegaly.

The clinical picture points to the diagnosis and in 90% of cases anti-nuclear factor is positive. The presence of antibodies to double-stranded DNA is diagnostic. Serum compliment in particular C3 and C4 are low. LE cells are usually present. Treatment is symptomatic, e.g. analgesics for joint involvement as well as high-dose steroids and other immunosuppressive therapy in active cases. The disease progresses with remissions and relapses. The 5-year survival rate is over 90%.

---

*E. Libman (1872–1946) American physician.
†B. Sacks (1873–1939). American physician.

Questions

A 73-year-old woman complained of tiredness, constipation, weight gain and tingling in her hands and feet. Investigations were as follows:

- Haemoglobin 10.0 g/dL
- White cell count 6×10^9/L
- MCV 101 fL
- Sodium 128 mmol/L
- Potassium 3.8 mmol/L
- Urea 6.0 mmol/L
- Random blood sugar 6.3 mmol/L
- Calcium 2.6 mmol/L
- Albumin 41 g/L
- fasting lipids – cholesterol 8.1 mmol/L
- Triglycerides 3.0 mmol/L
- Chest X-ray – cardiomegaly
- ECG – small complexes.

a. What is the most likely underlying diagnosis?
b. Explain the chest X-ray and ECG findings.
c. What is the most likely reason for the symptoms she has in her extremeties?

Answers

a. Hypothyroidism.

b. Percardial fluid is present. Pericardial effusions are very common in hypothyroidism and classically produce cardiomegaly with a 'pear-shaped' heart shadow. A pericardial effusion is also one of the causes of small QRS complexes on the ECG. There is a reduced amplitude of complexes in hypothyroidism even in the absence of a pericardial effusion. Other causes of small complexes include obesity and emphysema.

c. The most likely cause for the tingling in her hands and feet is a peripheral neuropathy due to B_{12} deficiency. She most likely has an associated pernicious anaemia that is a related autoimmune disease as she has a macrocytic anaemia. She may also be experiencing tingling in her hands due to carpal tunnel syndrome, which is also more common in patients with hypothryroidism.

Discussion

Hypothyroidism is more common in women and there is often a family history or a history of associated autoimmune diseases, e.g. pernicious anaemia. The onset is usually insidious and symptoms include: tiredness, weight gain, constipation, dry skin, croaky voice, cold intolerance, symptoms of carpal tunnel syndrome. There is often a typical facial appearance that includes peri-orbital oedema, facial puffiness, dry skin and a 'peaches and cream' complexion. The cream of the complexion is due to the associated anaemia and the peaches due to a hypercarotonaemia. There is a bradycardia and classically slow relaxation of the ankle jerks due to myotonia because of mucopolysaccharide infiltration of the muscles. There is a high incidence of ischaemic heart disease. Patients are often slow with intellectual impairment and dementia (myxoedema madness) can occur but is uncommon. Coma can also occur and hypothermia is more common.

Serum T4 is reduced and TSH is raised in an effort to stimulate a failing thyroid gland. Cholesterol is usually elevated. Hyponatraemia in this case can occur due to haemodilution. Anaemia may be normochromic or macrocytic. Hypothyroidism per se can cause macrocytosis as can B_{12} deficiency, which may be associated. Thyroid autoantibodies are often present. The ECG shows bradycardia with low amplitude complexes and there may be ST segment depression and T-wave inversion.

Treatment is with thyroxine, which is initially given in small doses (25 mcg for 1 month) and increased by 25 mcg daily every month until an adequate maintenance dose is reached (100–300 mcg daily). It is important to introduce the thyroxine slowly as its sympathomimetic effects can precipitate angina and tachyarrhythmias, particularly in the elderly.

Case histories

Questions

A 35-year-old woman complained of a 'flu-like' illness and a cough. She did not respond to a course of amoxycillin given by her GP. She complained of frontal headaches 2 weeks later and had had a nose bleed. On examination she was pyrexial (38°C) and dyspnoeic. She had a purpuric rash on her legs and a right foot drop. The results of investigations were:

- Chest X-ray – cavitating lesion right upper lobe and nodular shadow left lower lobe
- Full blood count – haemoglobin 10.8 g/dL normochromic/normocytic
- ESR 84 mm/h
- Urine – blood ++ protein ++.

a. What is the diagnosis?
b. List two further investigations that will help you confirm this.
c. What is the treatment?

Answers

(a) *Wegener's granulomatosis.

(b) 1. Open lung biopsy of the nodule in left lower lobe. Tissue biopsy is essential. Lesions in the nose can be biopsied. Biopsy characteristically shows multi-nucleated giant cells with necrotising vasculitis and granulomas.

    2. Cytoplasmic anti-neutrophil cytoplasm antibody (c-ANCA) estimation.

(c) Combination prednisolone (60 mg/od) and cyclophosphamide.

Discussion

Wegener's granulomatosis is a granulomatous, necrotising vasculitis involving the upper and lower respiratory tract producing epistaxis, sinusitis and destruction of the nasal cartilage (saddle nose). There are pulmonary nodules and diffuse infiltrates. This leads to cough, chest pain, dyspnoea and haemoptysis. The kidney is often involved resulting in glomerulonephritis and renal failure. Other systems may be involved. The frequency of involvement is as follows: respiratory tract (92%), kidney (85%), musculoskeletal system (67%), eye/orbit (52%), skin (46%), peripheral nervous system (15%), central nervous system (8%). The patient most commonly presents with fever, malaise, respiratory symptoms and a migratory arthritis. The disease affects females and males equally and most commonly presents in adulthood.

    Vasculitis of capillaries results in thrombosis and occlusion of the blood vessel lumen, which leads to necrosis. This and granulomatous infiltration are the histopathological hallmarks of the disease. The granulomatous formation may mimic mycobacterial and fungal infection, which should be excluded.

    The serum contains antibodies reacting with the cytoplasm of human neutrophils (c-ANCA) in 90% of patients with Wegener's granulomatosis. The target antigen for c-ANCA is a serine proteinase referred to as proteinase-3. Peri-nuclear ANCA (p-ANCA) is found in patients with crescentic glomerulonephritis whether or not in association with Wegener's granulomatosis so c-ANCA is more sensitive for Wegener's granulomatosis. However, in the absence of renal disease in Wegener's granulomatosis the sensitivity of c-ANCA is reduced to 70% of cases. False positives occur in infective and neoplastic disorders and therefore it is essential to get a tissue diagnosis.

If Wegener's granulomatosis is untreated the mean survival rate is 5 months. Treatment with combination oral prednisolone and low daily dose of cyclophosphamide improves survival. However, cyclophosphamide is associated with serious long-term toxic effects (bladder carcincoma, sterility, cystitis, myelodysplasia). Monthly high dose cyclophosphamide is less effective than low-dose daily regimes but less toxic. Other therapies (azathioprine and cyclosporin) have been shown to be less effective. Isolated sinus disease can be treated with saline irrigation. Arthralgia and arthritis is treated symptomatically with non-steroidal anti-inflammatory drugs.

---

*F. Wegener (born 1907). German pathologist.

Questions

A 52-year-old businessman complained of increasing breathlessness and palpitations. He had a cough productive of mucoid sputum. He denied having chest pain or haemoptysis. He was a non-smoker. His sister had a history of thyrotoxicosis. On examination he was slightly icteric and had finger clubbing. His heart rate was 140 b.p.m. and there were bilateral basal crackles on auscultation of his chest. His JVP (jugular venous pressure) was 4 cm and there was no peripheral oedema. His ECG confirmed atrial fibrillation and his chest X-ray showed pulmonary oedema. His thyroid function tests and random blood sugar were normal.

Full blood count showed:

- Haemoglobin 12.6 g/dL
- MCV 104 fL
- platelets 300×10^9
- White cell count 8.1×10^9/L

His liver function tests were as follows:

- ALT 140 IU/L
- Gamma GT 500 IU/L.

His echocardiogram showed a dilated left ventricle and an ejection fraction of 24%.
There was functional mitral regurgitation.

a. What treatment would you prescribe?
b. What is the most likely underlying aetiology?

Answers

a. Frusemide, digoxin (inotropic agent that also controls the ventricular rate). An ACE inhibitor should be introduced when his condition is more stable to reduce the morbidity and mortality associated with systolic dysfunction. If there are no contraindications he should receive full anti-coagulation with warfarin to reduce thromboembolic phenomenon and elective cardioversion should be considered.

b. Alcoholic cardiomyopathy (icteric, clubbed, macrocytosis). Clearly anticoagulation in this man would be a risk in view of his alcoholism and disturbed liver function.

Discussion

The patient had evidence of left ventricular failure. The fast ventricular rate could have precipitated this but he also had evidence of systolic dysfunction. However, echocardiographic measurement of ejection fraction is inaccurate with a rapid ventricular rate in this case although systolic function can be estimated from the two-dimensional images. It is better to repeat the echocardiogram when the ventricular rate is controlled. The history excluded thyrotoxicosis and there is nothing to suggest diabetes, ischaemic heart disease or valvular heart disease as the underlying aetiology. The macrocytosis and abnormal liver function tests as well as the echocardiogram add up to alcoholic cardiomyopathy. His profession may predispose to this (high levels of stress and business lunches with clients involving alcohol consumption).

Causes of congestive or dilated cardiomyopathy include: viral infection, ischaemic heart disease, hypertension, autoimmune disease, thyrotoxicosis and an inherited gene (rare, X-linked). There is progressive dilatation of both ventricles with functional valve regurgitation. Mural thrombosis is common and patients are at risk of systemic and pulmonary emboli. Cardiac arrhythmias are particularly common in alcoholic cardiomyopathy (atrial fibrillation and ventricular tachycardia). Treatment is symptomatic and withdrawal from alcohol is essential. Mitral valve replacement can be considered if mitral regurgitation is severe. Cardiac transplantation is the only hope of long-term survival in the young.

Questions

A 26-year-old man was brought to casualty after he had had a grand mal convulsion at work 2 hours previously. On examination he was drowsy but able to answer questions. He was unable to move his left arm and his reflexes were increased on the left with an extensor plantar response. He had a scoliosis and his blood pressure was 180/110 and pulse 70 b.p.m. Fundoscopy showed some retinal haemorrhages but no papilloedema. ECG showed left ventricular hypertrophy. He had had a spontaneous pneumothorax when he was 18 years old and learning difficulties as a child but there was no other significant history of note.

a. What is the probable cause of his fit?
b. How can his neurological signs be accounted for?
c. What is the cause of his abnormal ECG?
d. What is the underlying diagnosis?

Answers

a. A meningioma.

b. Localised paralysis, dysphasia, sensory disturbances, monoparesis or hemiparesis can occur after a fit and may last for a few hours (*Todd's paralysis). The signs may also be due to pressure from the meningioma in the right cerebral hemisphere.

c. His ECG indicates longstanding hypertension. Hypertension can occur after a fit but his blood pressure was high 2 hours later, which is unusual. Fundoscopy also indicates longstanding hypertension. Hypertension is a feature of raised intracranial pressure (secondary to the meningioma) but there were no other signs of this (bradycardia or papilloedema). Hypertension in this case is secondary (pheochromocytoma, renal artery stenosis).

d. Neurofibromatosis (†von Recklinghausen disease).

Discussion

Neurofibromatosis is one of the most common autosomal dominant disorders affecting 20 people in 100 000. It was described by von Recklinghausen in 1882. There are two distinct forms of this disease: von Recklinghausen (peripheral) neurofibromatosis and bilateral acoustic (central) neurofibromatosis. In the peripheral form the major features are: multiple café au lait spots, peripheral neurofibromas and Lisch nodules (pigmented iris hamartomas best seen with a split lamp). Other features include:

- Epilepsy
- Aqueduct stenosis
- Meningiomas
- Spinal neurofibromas
- Scoliosis (5% as in this case)
- Intellectual handicap (10% as in this case)
- Pseudoarthrosis (3%)
- Gastrointestinal fibromas (2%)
- Endocrine tumours (2% – especially pheochromocytosis, possibly in this case)
- Renal artery stenosis (2% – possibly in this case)
- Lung cysts (may result in spontaneous pneumothorax as in this case)
- Hamartomas of the retina
- Rib notching.

In central disease the main features are: bilateral acoustic neuromas and tumours of the central nervous system, especially meningiomas. Cutaneous lesions are uncommon and Lisch nodules are not seen. The central form of this disease is linked to abnormalities on chromosome 22.

---

*R.B. Todd (1809–1860). Irish physician.
†F.D. von Recklinghausen (1833–1910). Professor of pathology, Strasbourg.

Questions

A 50-year-old man collapsed while walking to the newsagent. He had been unemployed for 25 years following the onset of schizophrenia. His mental symptoms had been well controlled for 5 years. He was a heavy smoker. On examination he was confused and pale, and was generally hypotonic and weak. His blood pressure was 110/70 and heart rate 88 b.p.m. He was apyrexial and there was bronchial breathing at the right base. His blood results were as follows:

- Sodium 105 mmol/L
- Potassium 5.0 mmol/L
- Urea 1.3 mmol/L
- Total protein 40 g/L
- Albumin 26 g/L
- Calcium 2.7 mmol/L
- Haemoglobin 14.8 g/dL
- White cell count 16×10^9/L.

a. Give two possible explanations for his electrolyte abnormalities.
b. What is his corrected calcium level?
c. What is the treatment?

Answers

a. There is evidence of haemodilution (low sodium, low urea and low total protein). The most likely cause is inappropriate ADH secretion secondary to pneumonia and it is likely he has an underlying bronchial carcinoma (oat cell carcinoma, which secretes ADH) as he is a smoker. Another cause of inappropriate ADH secretion in this patient could be drugs, e.g. chlorpromazine used to treat his psychosis.

b. His corrected calcium is 2.98 mmol/L. He may have hypercalcaemia related to an underlying bronchial carcinoma secreting a parathyroid-like hormone (squamous cell carcinoma of the bronchus) or he may have bony metastases.

c. Treatment includes adequate investigations and initially the following tests should be organised: chest X-ray, ECG, random blood sugar, thyroid function tests, blood and urine osmolarity and arterial blood gases. He should be treated with i.v. saline and i.v. antibiotics. He should preferably receive hypertonic saline and he may require a forced diuresis (6 litres of i.v. fluid with i.v. frusemide) to reduce the serum calcium level initially. His electrolytes and fluid balance should be closely monitored. He would best be managed on a high dependency or intensive care unit in the first 24–48 hours.

Discussion

Hyponatraemia is the most frequent electrolyte disturbance seen in hospital and has an incidence of 1%. It may be asymptomatic and benign but it can however, cause brain damage, which is most commonly seen in children and young females. Cerebral oedema occurs in severe hyponatraemia, which leads to decreased cerebral blood flow and pressure necrosis. Tentorial herniation can occur with respiratory arrest, cerebral hypoxia and ischaemia.

The most common cause of hyponatraemia is probably postoperative when there is increased ADH secretion due to trauma, pain, stress, vomiting, sedatives or anaesthesia. ADH is produced by the hypothalmus and is stored in the posterior pituitary. It is usually released when vascular osmoreceptors are stimulated when it causes changes in the permeability of the collecting duct in the kidney and water is retained. Postoperative fluid prescription, if hypotonic, will contribute to hyponatraemia. Causes of inappropriate ADH secretion that produce hyponatraemia include: malignancy (bronchus, pancreas, Hodgkin's disease), infections (meningitis, pneumonia, tuberculosis), head injury, acute intermittent porphyria and drugs (chlorpromazine, carbamazepine). Other causes of hyponatraemia are: water overload, salt depletion (diarrhoea and vomiting), renal failure and hypothyroidism. AIDS is a major cause of hyponatraemia. It may be secondary to inappropriate ADH secretion or due to pulmonary or intracranial lesions, or to mineralocorticoid deficiency with intact glucocorticoid secretion (as AIDS affects the zona glomerulosa).

Treatment includes removing the underlying cause if possible. Asymptomatic hyponatraemia does not require aggressive management. Fluid restriction to < 1 L/d will increase sodium levels. Symptomatic hyponatraemia producing signs of encephalopathy requires urgent treatment to reduce cerebral oedema. Hypertonic saline should be given. In those with inappropriate ADH secretion there is a risk of circulatory overload and frusemide should be given simultaneously. Central venous pressure monitoring is essential. The plasma sodium should increase by 1 mmol/L/h and reach 130 mmol/L before stopping i.v. hypertonic saline. It has previously been suggested that rapid correction of hyponatraemia can lead to the development of a rare neurological syndrome called 'central pontine myelinolysis'. It is now known that rapid correction can lead to hypoxia and infarction causing neurological symptoms but usually rapid correction is not associated with significant morbidity or mortality. Central pontine myelinolysis is usually associated with patients with advanced liver disease, alcoholism, extensive burns, sepsis or malignancy who may also have hyponatraemia.

Questions

A 25-year-old woman complained of progressive dyspnoea on exertion for 6 months, weakness and dizziness. She had never been abroad and had been fit and well until now. She was taking no medication. On examination she was centrally cyanosed. Her pulse was 88 b.p.m. and irregular, and blood pressure 110/70 with a JVP of +6 cm. On auscultation there was a loud second heart sound and a pansystolic murmur heard best at the left sternal edge. Chest examination was normal. Her ECG showed right bundle branch block. T-wave inversion in leads V1–V4 and a QRS frontal axis of +120°.

a. What is the cause of her physical signs?
b. Name the most probable underlying diagnosis.

Answers

a. Pulmonary hypertension. She would also have a prominent 'a' wave in the JVP and a right ventricular (left parasternal) heave. Third and fourth heart sounds may also be present.

b. In order of probability the possible diagnoses are:

- Primary pulmonary hypertension
- Chronic pulmonary emboli (especially if she is taking the contraceptive pill)
- Congenital causes, e.g. atrial septal defect, ventricular septal defect, patent ductus arteriosis
- Cardiomyopathy
- Other causes of pulmonary hypertension, e.g. aortic valve disease, mitral valve disease, ischaemic heart disease, chronic obstructive pulmonary disease, pulmonary fibrosis (these would not fit with this history).

Discussion

Primary pulmonary hypertension is rare but is more common in young women. There is an association with Raynaud's phenomenon and hepatic cirrhosis. The condition is usually fatal within 3 years and the only hope of long-term survival is a heart–lung transplant. Patients should be given anti-coagulation medication. Some drugs lower pulmonary artery pressure. Nifedipine and diltiazem have been used with limited success. Intravenous prostacyclin (epoprostenol) is expensive but can be used intermittently to lower pulmonary artery pressure. Spontaneous improvement may occur but this is rare.

Questions

A 23-year-old man complained of a 1-week history of flu-like illness, fatigue and polyarthritis. On examination his temperature was 38°C and his respiratory rate was 18 breaths per minute. His heart rate was 100 b.p.m. and blood pressure 110/70. There were no other abnormalities on examination. He had never been ill before and worked as a gardener. Investigation results were as follows:

- Haemoglobin 12.8 g/dL
- White cell count 14×10^9/L
- Sodium 140 mmol/L
- Potassium 3.5 mmol/L
- Urea 10 mmol/L
- Random blood sugar 4.1 mmol/L
- Chest X-ray – bilateral upper lobe shadowing
- ECG – sinus tachycardia.

a. What is the diagnosis?
b. Name one investigation to confirm this diagnosis.
c. What is the treatment?

Answers

a. Mycoplasma pneumonia. Legionnaires' disease is unlikely as the patient is usually sicker with diarrhoea, myalgia and confusion and the lung bases are more commonly affected. Pulmonary aspergillosis is a possibility but this would more commonly occur in the immuno-suppressed. However, gardeners are more susceptible as they are exposed to aspergillus in the soil.

b. A rise in mycoplasma antibodies in the serum in a convalescent sample. The organism may be isolated from the sputum but one-third of cases have no sputum. Cold agglutinins to type O human red cells are usually present.

c. Tetracycline or erythromycin.

Discussion

Mycoplasma pneumoniae (Eaton agent) is the only pathogenic mycoplasma known to man. It has its highest incidence in winter and occurs in four yearly epidemic cycles (1996 was the last epidemic year). Children and young adults are most commonly affected. The radiological features may be dramatic and be out of proportion to the clinical picture. A 'flu-like' illness often precedes polymyalgia, anorexia and malaise and this is followed by respiratory symptoms. Full recovery is usual.

Questions

A 60-year-old man was admitted with acute dypsnoea. On examination his pulse was 120 and irregular and blood pressure 120/70, JVP + 6 cm and there were bilateral crackles on chest auscultation. He had a grey colouration of his skin, gynaecomastia and finger clubbing. There was evidence of hepatomegaly. He was a lifelong non-smoker and non-drinker. He had been taking the following drugs for 6 months: frusemide 40 mg/d and amiodarone 200 mg/d. His urgent investigations were as follows:

- Sodium 130 mmol/L
- Potassium 3.9 mmol/L
- Urea 12.7 mmol/L
- Random blood sugar 17.1 mmol/L
- Chest X-ray – pulmonary oedema
- ECG – atrial fibrillation.

a. What is the underlying diagnosis?
b. Give two possible reasons for his skin discolouration.

Answers

a. Haemochromatosis.

b. Haemosiderin deposition associated with haemochromatosis. Amiodarone can also cause a slate grey discolouration of the skin.

Discussion

Haemochromatosis is more common in men and is inherited as an autosomal recessive condition. It is associated with *HLA-A3* and *HLA-B7*. It presents in men at any age but in women only after the menopause (physiological bleeding results in protection). It is due to excessive iron absorption, which is deposited in the tissues – usually liver, pancreas, heart, synovial membranes and endocrine glands.

Clinically the patient is diabetic (in 80% of cases) and has brown (due to melonin) or slate grey (due to haemosiderin) pigmentation of the skin, (hence the term 'bronze diabetes'). There is hepatomegaly and cirrhosis. Signs of chronic liver disease may be present: testicular atrophy, gynaecomastia, loss of body hair, finger clubbing, Dupuytren's contracture etc. Pseudogout particularly affects the wrist, hips and knees and is common (40% of cases). Cardiac infiltration results in a restrictive cardiomyopathy with congestive heart failure and arrhythmias a common presentation. Hepatocellular carcinoma occurs in 30% of cases if untreated.

The diagnosis is confirmed by a high serum ferritin level and iron levels. Treatment consists of weekly venesection (500 ml) until the serum ferritin is < 10 µg/L. This takes 2–3 years and then maintenance venesection is required every 2–3 months.

Questions

A 32-year-old woman complained of fatigue, anorexia and weight loss for 1 week and photophobia for 24 h, which was accompanied by painful erythematous lesions on her arms. Her twin sister, who she had seen 10 days previously, complained of similar symptoms and developed left facial palsy and neck stiffness but there was no other family history of note.

Full blood count and electrolytes were normal and corrected serum calcium was 2.9 mmol/L. A chest X-ray showed non-specific basal shadowing. Her ECG showed first-degree heart block and complete right bundle branch block.

a. What is the most likely diagnosis?
b. What are the lesions on her arms?
c. Name two other causes of these lesions.
d. What is the cause of the hypercalcaemia?

Answers

a. Sarcoidosis – more common in families and a genetic link has been proposed as has an infective agent. Meningitis is an unlikely diagnosis in this case, the cause of the photophobia being anterior uveitis. Neck stiffness is due to meningeal involvement. The differential diagnosis includes: Wegener's granulomatosis and some infections that can produce a similar picture (histoplasmosis, tuberculosis).

b. Erythema nodosum. Histologically this is not sarcoid but shows subcutaneous inflammatory change that is vasculitic.

c. Causes of erythema nodosum include: streptococcal infections, tuberculosis, syphilis, toxoplasmosis, fungal infection, inflammatory bowel disease, pregnancy, rheumatic fever, Behçet's disease, drugs (sulphonamides, penicillin, oral contraceptive pill, salicylates).

d. This is due to an overproduction of 1,25-dihydroxy vitamin D, which increases calcium absorption and bone resorption. Bone cysts can occur and this produces a risk of nephrolithiasis and renal failure.

Discussion

Sarcoidosis is a systemic disorder of varying severity. It is more common in females (5:1), non-Caucasians, Irish and Scandinavians. It usually occurs in the young (< 40 years old). The pathological hallmark is a non-caseating granuloma. The aetiology is unknown but often a known cause of granulomatous inflammation may be found, e.g. chronic beryllium disease. Community outbreaks suggest that the disease is spread from person to person via an antigen or environmental agent. Genetic factors may play a role in a predisposed host who produces an exaggerated cellular immune response. Sarcoidosis is more common in monozygotic than dizygotic twins and familial clusters occur. Some association has been found with HLA-38 *HLA1-B8* and *-DR3*.

The clinical presentation is usually of systemic upset. The onset may be acute or chronic. Up to 50% of individuals affected have features of *Lofgrens' syndrome: erythema nodosum, hilar lymphadenopathy and acute iritis. Other clinical features are:

1. **Respiratory** – occurs in nearly all cases. May present as asymptomatic bilateral hilar lymphadenopathy on the chest X-ray. Pulmonary fibrosis is a common feature but chronic airflow limitation can also occur due to lobar stenosis, which can mimic asthma. There may be sinus disease and palatal destruction.

2. **Cardiovascular** – serious cardiac dysfunction occurs in 5–10%. Papillary dysfunction, infiltrative cardiomyopathy and pericarditis can occur.

3. **Nervous system** – facial palsy is the most common presentation (may be bilateral). Meningeal irritation and peripheral neuropathy occur in 3%.

4. **Endocrine/biochemical** – there is increased serum calcium, angiotensin converting enzyme and globulins.

5. **Eyes** – 25% of cases are affected. Iritis and anterior uveitis cause blurred vision, photophobia and can cause blindness. Conjunctival involvement with yellow nodules is common.

6. **Skin** – erythema nodosum, plaques and nodules sometimes occur in scars, lupus pernio (violaceous lesions on nose and cheeks, lips and ears). Lupus pernio has a predilection for women, especially Negroid women.

7. **Miscellaneous** – parotitis, hepatosplenomegaly, bone cysts, generalised lymphadenopathy.

Diagnosis is clinical. It is important to biopsy tissue. Skin and trans-bronchial biopsies give the most information and a liver biopsy may be helpful if there is liver involvement, but this is not without risk. Kveim testing shows false-negative reactions in 25% of cases and is not always useful. Treatment is symptomatic if symptoms are mild due to a high possibility of spontaneous improvement. Systemic corticosteroids are indicated for severe ocular, neurological and cardiorespiratory disease, and hypercalcaemia. Prognosis is better for young persons, if the onset is more acute and if there is bilateral hilar lymphadenopathy alone without other respiratory involvement. The condition may recur.

*S. Lofgren. Swedish physician.

Question

A 72-year-old man complained that he had had three blackouts in the previous month. On one occasion he had sustained a fractured nose and clavicle. The blackouts occurred without warning and usually when he was walking outdoors. His wife was with him on one occasion and said he suddenly fell to the ground and was unrousable for 2 minutes. He did not move and looked pale. On regaining consciousness he felt quite alert. He had been taking bendrofluazide 2.5 mg daily for 10 years for hypertension but there was no other past medical history of note. He smoked 10 cigarettes a day.

On examination his heart rate was 64 b.p.m. sinus rhythm and blood pressure 120/80 with no postural drop. He had a systolic murmur and a right carotid bruit. His ECG showed left bundle branch block and a chest X-ray was normal.

a. Give two possible causes of his blackouts.

Answers

1. Aortic stenosis – this may be significant as his blood pressure was low with a narrow pulse pressure and there was evidence of left ventricular strain (left bundle branch block).

2. Arrhythmia – this may be secondary to valve disease or ischaemic heart disease. His risk factors for ischaemic heart disease are hypertension and smoking and there was clinical evidence of vascular disease (right carotid bruit).

Discussion

The cause of his blackouts is most likely cardiac syncope. They are significant as indicated by substantial injury. It is unlikely he has had a fit as he was motionless when he fell suddenly with no warning and he felt alert after the event. Although he has a carotid bruit the blackout is not likely to be a transient ischaemic attack as these are almost never a cause of loss of consciousness. The presence of a bruit indicates vascular disease but there is no correlation between its presence and carotid artery stenosis. Investigation must include a 24-hour ECG and echocardiogram. Significant aortic stenosis, which is symptomatic (dyspnoea, syncope, angina) carries a significant mortality with an average survival of 18 months to 3 years. 24-hour ECG may need to be repeated or an 8-day event recorder may be more useful in this case.

Other cardiac causes of syncope include hypotensive episodes (due to bendrofluazide) and carotid sinus hypersensitivity. Carotid sinus syndrome has been implicated in 14% of those over 65-year-olds suffering syncope. The syndrome is due to hypersensitivity of the baroreceptor cells in the carotid sinus located at the bifurcation of the common carotid artery. Symptoms of syncope, falls or dizziness may occur and be provoked by neck movements. There are two types of carotid sinus syndrome: cardioinhibitory, when carotid sinus massage causes at least a 3 s asystolic pause and vasodepressor, when carotid sinus massage causes a fall in systolic blood pressure of at least 50 mmHg. Approximately one-third of cases are cardioinhibitory in type, one-third are vasodepressor and one-third are mixed types (both cardioinhibitory and vasodepressor). Carotid sinus massage would be contraindicated in this patient because of the presence of a carotid bruit, which may result in provoking cerebrovascular symptoms. Treatment of cardioinhibitory carotid sinus syndrome is a permanent dualchamber pacemaker but the treatment of the vasodepressor type is less satisfactory. Hypotensive agents, e.g. nitrates and ACE inhibitor drugs should be discontinued if possible. Fludrocortisone and ephedrine may be necessary to improve symptoms.

Questions

A 70-year-old woman was found drowsy and confused at home by her son. She had complained in recent weeks of constipation and also that her eyes were troubling her in that she had altered colour perception. Her son who was diabetic said she was normally well except she had attended a hospital nuclear medicine department appointment 6 months previously but he did not know the details of this.

On examination she looked pale, and was drowsy and disorientated. Her pulse was 38 b.p.m. and irregular and her blood pressure was 150/80. Her heart sounds were only just audible but normal. There were no focal neurological signs. Investigations were as follows:

- Chest X-ray normal
- ECG – slow atrial fibrillation
- Full blood count – haemoglobin 9.6 g/dL
- MCV 101 fL
- Platelets 100×10^9/L
- White cell count 3.1×10^9/L
- Random blood sugar 7.6 mmol/L
- INR 3.0
- Urea 7 mmol/L
- Sodium 138 mmol/L
- Potassium 3.0 mmol/L.

a. Name two reasons for her current clinical state?
b. What is the cause of her anaemia?
c. Why did she attend the nuclear medicine department 6 months previously?

Answers

a. Hypothyroidism – confusion, drowsiness, slow atrial fibrillation, constipation. Digoxin toxicity – slow atrial fibrillation, altered colour vision, constipation.

b. Pernicious anaemia – there is an association with thyroid disease. She has a typical picture of macrocytosis and suppression of white blood cells and platelets as seen in megaloblastic anaemias.

c. She attended for radio-iodine therapy for thyrotoxicosis. Up to 25% of patients develop hypothyroidism 3–6 months later. She probably had rapid atrial fibrillation associated with thyrotoxicosis and was taking digoxin to control the ventricular rate and warfarin to reduce thromboemboli associated with atrial fibrillation.

Discussion

This woman most likely had Grave's disease and had radio-iodine treatment. This is an auntoimmune disease and is associated with other autoimmune diseases: diabetes mellitus, pernicious anaemia, Addison's disease, hypoparathyroidism, myasthenia gravis, systemic sclerosis. There is a genetic propensity (her son has diabetes) and there is a relationship with *HLA-B8* and *DR3*.

She may well also have had digoxin toxicity as patients with hypothyroidism become sensitive to the effects of digoxin whereas conversely thyrotoxicosis results in digoxin resistance. Features of digoxin toxicity include: anorexia, nausea, vomiting, diarrhoea, malaise, fatigue, confusion, facial pain, insomnia, depression, disordered colour vision known as xanthopsia (green or yellow halos around objects and lights), arrhythmias that may be bradycardias or supraventricular tachycardia or ventricular tachycardia. Digoxin is mainly excreted via the kidneys (80%) and only partly by the liver (20%). Impaired renal function will result in digoxin toxicity. Other situations in which there may be a sensitivity to digoxin include: hypokalaemia, hypomagnesaemia, hypercalcaemia, acute myocardial infarction and interactions with other drugs, e.g. verapamil, diltiazem hydrochloride, beta-blockers, amiodarone. Some antibiotics, e.g. erythromycin also increase levels of digoxin and therefore result in toxicity as they destroy the bacteria that convert digoxin into inactive products in the gut, resulting in an increased absorption of digoxin. Digoxin is now more widely used not only to control the ventricular rate in patients with atrial fibrillation but also as an inotropic agent in congestive heart failure, even in the presence of sinus rhythm. It has been found to prevent the worsening of heart failure in such cases and also reduce hospitalisation but it has not had any effect on the mortality associated with heart failure. Treatment of digoxin toxicity is symptomatic and involves withdrawal of the drug. Digibind (specific digoxin antibodies) can also be used in severe cases of digoxin toxicity but the drug is expensive and there is an incidence of allergic reactions.

Questions

A 29-year-old woman complained of increased clumsiness, pains in her shoulders and falls for 1 week. She had a history of epilepsy and had had an upper respiratory tract infection 2 weeks previously but was otherwise well. She had not had childhood vaccinations as her mother had refused these because of her epilepsy.

On examination she had a peripheral neuropathy and weakness of both legs with decreased tone and absent reflexes. She had bilateral VIIth cranial nerve lesions. Her investigations were as follows:

- Full blood count – haemoglobin 13.1 g/dL
- White cell count 3.9×10^9/L
- Random blood sugar 6.1 mmol/L
- Electrolytes normal
- ESR 10 mm/h.

a. What one investigation would you perform?
b. What is the diagnosis?

Answers

a. Lumbar puncture.
b. Acute postinfective polyneuropathy *Guillain–†Barre syndrome).

Discussion

The symptoms usually follow a flu-like illness: they are sensory and motor, the latter usually predominating. There may be a glove and stocking neuropathy or sensation may be affected in patches. Paralysis usually occurs distally and moves proximally with a flaccid picture and loss of reflexes. Sphincter control is usually preserved. Dysphagia can occur as well as cerebellar and upper motor neurone signs. Cardiac arrhythmias may be a feature. Pains in the shoulder and back are common. Facial and ocular muscles are often affected. Facial palsy (usually lower motor neurone) when unilateral is easier to detect due to the asymmetry. Bilateral facial palsies are more difficult to detect and have other causes: bilateral Bell's palsy, myasthenia gravis, motor neurone disease, muscular dystrophy, sarcoidosis, mononeuritis multiplex. When the respiratory muscles are involved in the polyneuritis, ventilation may be needed. The ‡Miller Fisher syndrome is thought to be a variant of Guillian–Barré and is characterised by ophthalmoplegia, ataxia and areflexia.

The diagnosis is clinical and is confirmed by the characteristic lumbar puncture findings of a high protein concentration in the CSF fluid (30–100 g/l) with few white cells and normal sugar concentration. The differential diagnosis to be considered is poliomyelitis but this does not affect the sensory nerves and is usually asymmetrical with CSF showing lower protein and raised white cells. The absence of immunisation in this case is pointing to this diagnosis being considered. The relatively low white cell count is indicative of a recent or current viral infection.

Management is supportive. The patient's nutrition and fluid balance should be monitored. There is a risk of infection and thrombosis, especially if ventilation is required for respiratory failure and prophylactic heparin is indicated. Specific treatments, e.g. plasmapheresis can be of benefit. Recovery is usually complete but may take several months. Mortality is around 10%. The condition can recur in a small proportion of cases.

---

*C. Guillain (1876–1961). French neurologist.
†J.A. Barré (1886–1967). Professor of neurology.
‡Miller Fisher. Canadian neurologist.

Questions

A 27-year-old man presented with a painful swollen right knee and back-ache. He complained of malaise, anorexia and weight loss. He found it difficult to eat due to painful mouth ulcers. He had been to Morocco the month before on holiday. On examination he had a macular rash on his hands and feet, his temperature was 37.5°C and he looked pale. Investigations were as follows:

- Haemoglobin 10.1 g/dL
- MCV 98fL
- White cell count $7.8 \times 10^9/L$
- ESR 90 mm/h
- Chest X-ray normal.

a. What is the diagnosis?
b. What is the rash?
c. Why did he have backache?

Answers

a. *Reiter's disease.
b. Keratoderma blenorrhagica.
c. Sacroiliitis.

Discussion

Reiter's disease comprises of a classical triad of urethritis, conjunctivitis and arthritis following an enteric infection (usually shigella, salmonella, yersinia or Campylobacter) or genitourinary contact. However, in the UK most cases occur in males (10:1) in association with non-specific urethritis. HLA-B27 is found in 80% of cases and there may also be an association with HLA-B7, BW22 and BW42. The disease is less common in Negroes who seldom possess HLA-B27.

There is often systemic upset. The arthritis is seronegative, inflammatory, mono or oligo-arthritis, which most commonly affects the knees and ankles. Achilles tendonitis and plantar fasciitis are common as is sacroiliitis. Urethritis produces a sterile clear urethral discharge with minimal dysuria and it may be asymptomatic as in this case. There may be a haemorrhagic cystitis or prostatitis. Ocular involvement is usually mild bilateral conjunctivitis, which subsides in a few weeks. It may progress to episcleritis, anterior uveitis and corneal irritation. Mouth ulcers are common. Balanitis and keratoderma blenorrhagica are pathognomonic. Rarer manifestations are: pericariditis, pleurisy, pulmonary infiltrate, myocarditis, aortic regurgitation and peripheral neuropathy. The condition is self-limiting in 50% of cases. It can relapse and become chronic and 15% suffer permanent disability. Differential diagnosis of the arthritis includes gout, which it may mimic in the acute phase. Gonococcal arthritis can also produce similar features. Keratoderma blenorrhagica may sometimes be indistinguishable from pustular psoriasis. †Behçet's disease usually has painful genital ulcers and more severe eye involvement. The genital ulcers in Reiter's disease are painless.

Treatment is symptomatic. Occasionally systemic steroids may be needed and rarely cytotoxic drugs such as methotrexate.

---

*H.C. Reiter (1881–1961). German professor of hygiene.
†H. Behçet (1889–1948). Turkish dermatologist.

Questions

A 40-year-old man complained of repeatedly dropping small objects and having a swollen right elbow. He was a DIY fanatic and a heavy smoker. On examination he had a kyphoscoliosis and pectus excavatum. He had tar staining to his right finger and several healed scars on his hands. There was bilateral wasting of the small muscles of the hands with reduced sensation to pain. His right elbow was deformed and range of movement painless and reduced. He had a right *Horners' syndrome. There was increased tone in his legs and plantar responses were extensor.

a. What is the differential diagnosis?
b. What two investigations would you request?

Answers

a. Syringomyelia (an intermedullary tumour or haemorrhage – haemato-myelia) can give similar symptoms and signs). Carcinoma of lung (C6–C8 infiltration) is a possibility but does not usually produce Charcot's joints (painless and deformed), which implies chronicity of the condition.

b. MRI scan of the cervical and thoracic cord, CT scan of the chest and chest X-ray are all acceptable.

Discussion

Syringomyelia is a disease that results from a congenital longitudinal cyst in the cervical cord and/or brainstem anterior to the spinal cord. It spreads asymmetrically to each side. It may be associated with other con-genital abnormalities such as spina bifida and naevia over the vertebra. The fibres that cross in the mid-line (spinothalamic tracts) are particu-larly affected causing loss of pain and temperature sensation in the der-matomes affected on both sides of the body. Touch and proprioception, which are carried in the posterior columns are unaffected. This is 'disso-ciated' sensory loss – the anterior horn cells are commonly affected, giv-ing lower motor neurone weakness and wasting. Pressure on the pyramidal tracts causes a spastic paraparesis. Extension upwards into the medulla causes involvement of the trigeminal nerve as well as the bulbar motor nuclei (IX–XII), (syringobulbia) *Horner's syndrome may result from involvement of the sympathetic tract.

Other conditions causing wasting of the small muscles of the hand include: motor neurone disease, cervical spondylosis, Pancoast's tumour, cervical rib.

Treatment is by surgical decompression of the cyst.

---

*J.F. Horner (1831–1886). Swiss ophthalmologist

Questions

A 26-year-old woman complained of increasing exertional dyspnoea, which lasted over 6 months and recurrent chest infections. She had collapsed twice and regularly felt dizzy. On examination she was cyanosed and had finger clubbing. Her JVP was +8 cm, her heart rate 100 b.p.m. and her blood pressure 110/70. She had a parasternal heave and a loud second heart sound. She also had an ejection systolic murmur and an early diastolic murmur at the left sternal edge. There were bilateral basal crackles.

a. What is the most likely cause of the diastolic murmur?
b. What is the diagnosis?
c. Name two possible ECG abnormalities.

Answers

a. Pulmonary regurgitation (*Graham Steell murmur) due to pulmonary hypertension. Other signs of pulmonary hypertension are; parasternal heave, loud second heart sound, right ventricular fourth heart sound and pansystolic murmur due to tricuspid regurgitation. An apical mid diastolic murmur can sometimes be heard due to the increased flow through the mitral valve.

b. †Eisenmenger's syndrome – this refers to the reversal of a left to right shunt as a result of pulmonary hypertension. The usual congenital defects are: ventricular septal defect, patent ductus arteriosis and atrial septal defect.

c. Signs of right ventricular strain: right bundle branch block, right axis deviation, right ventricular hypertrophy.

Discussion (see case history 5)

This patient unfortunately presented too late, the congenital defect going undetected and resulting in a reversed shunt and Eisenmenger's syndrome. The most likely underlying congenital defect is a ventricular septal defect. The recurrent chest infections this patient has are secondary to pulmonary hypertension. It is unlikely she has bronchiectasis as the initial diagnosis (symptoms including: finger clubbing, pulmonary hypertension, cyanosis) and the history is too short. She has signs of cardiac failure (crackles, raised JVP, tachycardia) due to ventricular overload caused by the shunt. When Eisenmenger's syndrome has developed the cardiac shunt is irreparable and the only hope of cure is a heart–lung transplant. The patient experiences dizziness, angina, dyspnoea and syncope. Secondary polycythaemia occurs, which increases the risk of thrombosis and causes headaches, dizziness and pruritus. Regular venesection is necessary. Infections (particularly chest infections) and skin sepsis (acne is a problem) are typical features. Cerebral abscess is recognised as a problem with passage of bacteria across the shunt. Gout is common secondary to polycythaemia. Subacute bacterial endocarditis prophylaxis is necessary. Altitude should be avoided due to hypoxia. Contraception is poorly tolerated – the oral contraceptive pill increases the risk of thrombosis in these patients and intrauterine contraceptive devices carry a risk of infection.

---

*Graham Steell (1851–1942). Scottish physician.
†V. Eisenmenger (1864–1932). German physician.

Questions

A 70-year-old woman complained of a 2-week history of malaise, neck and shoulder pain and stiffness and low back pain. She had lost 4 kg in weight in 4 weeks due to anorexia. Her symptoms were worse in the morning. She had no past medical history of note. She had a sister with hypothyroidism and diabetes. On examination the range of movement of all joints was full but shoulder joint movement was painful. She had extensive *Heberden's and †Bouchard's nodes. Her blood results were as follows:

- Haemoglobin 10.4 g/dL
- MCV 88 fL
- Platelets $600 \times 10^9/L$
- Electrolytes normal
- ESR 76 mm/h.

a. What is the diagnosis?
b. Name a diagnostic test for this condition.
c. What is the treatment?

---

*W. Heberden (1710–1801). English physician.
†C.J. Bouchard (1837–1915). French physician.

Answers

a. Polymyalgia rheumatica. Hypothyroidism can cause similar symptoms but there is usually weight gain not weight loss and there may be a normochromic/normocytic anaemia; however, the ESR is usually normal in hypothyroidism. She also has osteoarthritis, which is longstanding (Heberden's and Bouchard's nodes).

b. A diagnostic test specific for polymyalgia rheumatica does not exist and the diagnosis is mainly clinical.

c. Prednisolone 10–15 mg daily for 4 weeks. The dose should then be reduced slowly and patients are usually maintained on a dose that controls symptoms for about 2 years. A dose of 7.5 mg/d or less should be achieved as at this dose the incidence of side-effects from prednisolone is much reduced.

Discussion

Polymyalgia rheumatica is more common in elderly women (> 60 years old; the female: male ratio 3:1). It is more common in Scandanavia, North America and the UK, and in Caucasians. It is characterised by proximal muscle pain and stiffness; there is no weakness. The onset is usually sudden and mainly affects the shoulders and upper arms but can affect the buttocks and thighs in a symmetrical manner. The muscles may be tender but there is no wasting. Movements may be limited by pain and stiffness but there is no weakness. Symptoms are usually worse in the morning. Associated systemic features include: malaise, weight loss, joint pain, and swelling and depression.

The diagnosis is clinical and there are no specific tests. The (ESR) is usually increased (> 40 mm/h). Alkaline phosphatase (liver origin) is increased in 30% of cases. There may be a normochromic/normocytic anaemia and a thrombocythaemia. The differential diagnoses to be considered and excluded are: late onset rheumatoid arthritis, other connective tissue disorders, hypothyroidism, multiple myeloma and polymyositis. Other clinical features in these conditions and other biochemical investigations will exclude them.

There is a close link with polymyalgia rheumatica and temporal arteritis. About 25% of patients with polymyalgia rheumatica also have temporal arteritis. In the latter there is a severe usually unilateral headache with tenderness of the scalp, especially over the temporal artery. There may be visual blurring and jaw claudication. Visual involvement is due to inflammation of the ophthalmic arteries causing retinal ischaemia and blindness can occur. Cerebral and coronary arteries can also be affected. Urgent treatment with high-dose steroids is needed to prevent visual loss (40–60 mg prednisolone o.d.). Temporal artery biopsy shows patchy involvement of the arterial wall with mononuclear and giant cells and areas of necrosis.

Treatment of polymyalgia rheumatica with steroids results in a rapid clinical response and the ESR usually falls within 3 weeks. Patients should be maintained on steroids for about 2 years and they should be advised to watch for symptoms of headaches and blurred vision. In some patients it is impossible to withdraw steroids and they usually remain on prednisolone 2–3 mg daily for life. Monitoring the patient should be based on the clinical picture as a priority rather than the ESR.

The prognosis is good and there is a low rate of recurrence of the condition after 2 years.

Questions

A 76-year-old man complained of a sudden onset of headache, diplopia and nausea of 2 hours' duration. He had had a myocardial infarction 10 years previously and after this he stopped smoking and took digoxin 250 mcg daily and aspirin 300 mg daily. He had had a partial gastrectomy 30 years previously for a duodenal ulcer but there was no other past history of note.

On examination he had a right partial ptosis and an abductive right eye with a dilated pupil. There was no neck stiffness and he was apyrexial. His heart rate was 88 b.p.m., he was in atrial fibrillation and his blood pressure was 200/90. His ECG showed atrial fibrillation and left ventricular hypertrophy. Other investigations were as follows:

- Haemoglobin 10.6 g/dL.
- MCV 86 fL
- White cell count 3.9×10^9/L
- Platelets 146×10^9/L
- Serum iron – low
- Total iron binding capacity – high
- Electrolytes – normal
- ESR 30 mm/h
- Random blood sugar 6.6 mmol/L.

a. Name three differential diagnoses.
b. What is the cause of his double vision?
c. List two possible causes of his anaemia.

Answers

a. • Subarachnoid haemorrhage
   • Embolic stroke (he is in atrial fibrillation)
   • Haemorrhage stroke (he is taking aspirin and has evidence of longstanding hypertension, i.e. left ventricular hypertrophy on his ECG).
   • Meningitis is unlikely in this case but should be considered.
   • Ophthalmoplegic migraine can cause similar symptoms but there is usually a past history beginning in childhood.

b. Right partial third cranial nerve palsy. He has partial ptosis and a divergent squint most likely due to a posterior communicating artery aneurysm. Other causes of a third cranial nerve palsy include:

1. Mononeuritis multiplex (diabetes mellitus, rheumatoid arthritis, sarcoidosis, amyloidosis, carcinoma, systemic lupus erythematosus, polyarteritis nodosum, Wegener's granulomatosis).

2. Mid-brain vascular lesion.

3. Mid-brain demyelination.

4. Ophthalmoplegic migraine.

5. Neoplasms (base of skull, sphenoidal wing meningioma).

6. Encephalitis.

c. Iron deficiency anaemia (due to aspirin-induced gastric erosions), B_{12} deficiency due to his previous partial gastrectomy. It is likely he has both as the MCV is normal in the presence of iron-studies confirming iron deficiency anaemia. A slightly suppressed white cell count and platelet count is associated with B_{12} deficiency.

Discussion

The most common cause of subarachnoid haemorrhage is rupture of a cerebral aneurysm (25% of cases have multiple aneurysms). It carries a mortality rate of 40–60% and a high morbidity. The classical presentation is of a sudden severe headache that may be accompanied by vomiting, collapse and loss of consciousness. Neck stiffness and photophobia may occur and there may be focal (cortical or cranial nerve) neurological deficit.

Initial investigations should include a non-contrast CT scan, which will reveal subarachnoid blood in more than 80% of cases. If the CT scan is not diagnostic a lumbar puncture should be performed. This should be done at least 12 h after the onset of the headache to allow time for the development of xanthochromia from red cell breakdown. If this is negative (in a small minority) cerebral angiography should be considered.

The morbidity and mortality from subarachnoid haemorrhage depends on the severity of the initial bleed, re-bleeding and cerebral ischaemia. The aim of treatment therefore is to prevent re-bleeding and secondary ischaemia. All patients should be referred to a neurosurgeon for consideration of early clipping of the aneurysm. All patients should receive active resuscitation with i.v. fluids and oxygen and vital parameters (blood pressure, pulse, venous pressure) should be monitored. Nimodipine (60 mg 4 hourly) has been shown to be well tolerated and reduce cerebral infarction; all patients should receive this. The timing of surgery is difficult but 70% of re-bleeds can be prevented by early surgery (within 4 days).

The prognosis after treatment including neurosurgical clipping is good but two-thirds of those who survive will have some neurological deficit and the remainder will be symptom free.

Questions

A 41-year-old man had a sore throat for 3 days and visited his GP, who pre-scribed amoxycillin 500 mg t.d.s. On the sixth day he developed rigors, a cough, painful eyes, mouth and joints.

On examination he was pyrexial at 38.5°C, had a cold sore on the upper lip and several aphthous ulcers in his mouth. There was a gener-alised erythematous rash mainly on his hands, arms and feet, which was maculopapular with one or two vesicles. Investigations were as follows:

- Haemoglobin 12.6 g/dL
- White cell count 16.1×10^9/L
- Urea 18.3 mmol/L
- Creatinine 162 mmol/L
- Potassium 4.1 mmol/L
- Sodium 150 mmol/L
- Chest X-ray – right basal opacity consistent with consolidation.

a. What is the dermatological diagnosis?
b. List three possible causes of this.

Answers

a. *†Stevens–Johnson syndrome. Erythema multiforme with mucosal ulceration and pyrexia.

b. Drug-induced (amoxycillin), streptococcal pneumonia (chest X-ray shows consolidation), Herpes simplex virus.

Discussion

Stevens–Johnson syndrome is the eruption of erythema multiforme associated with severe mucosal lesions (affecting eyes, mouth and genitalia) and systemic upset (fever, malaise, vomiting, joint pains, renal failure, diarrhoea and polyarthritis). The rash is also known by the more descriptive term 'erythema bullosum malignans'. The rash is symmetrical and usually affects the extremities more than the trunk. The lesions are erythematous, coin shaped and may coalesce. There is often blistering in the centre (target shaped lesions). The centre of the lesion is usually darker than the periphery. The erythema disappears with pressure and they are not itchy.

The aetiology is unknown in half of the cases. Other causes are:

1. Infections (herpes simplex, mycoplasma, streptococcus, typhoid, diphtheria)
2. Drugs (sulphonamides, penicillin, salicylate, quinine)
3. Neoplasia, DXT
4. Ulcerative colitis and Crohn's disease
5. Connective tissue disorders (rheumatoid arthritis, lupus erythematosus).

Treatment includes finding the cause and removing it. Steroids are used (prednisolone 40 mg daily). Secondary infection should be treated with appropriate antibiotics. In this case i.v. erythromycin may be used as the patient has pneumonia and it is not clear if amoxycillin has induced the skin condition. Appropriate microbiological investigations must be initiated before antibiotics are given, i.e. blood cultures, sputum culture, MSSU, throat swab, anti-streptolysin titre. Blood gases are essential. The patient requires close monitoring with i.v. fluids and the monitoring of renal and respiratory function.

The patients are usually extremely unwell and there is a significant risk of mortality. The condition may recur.

---

*A.M. Stevens (1884–1945). American paediatrician.
†F.C. Johnson (1894–1934). American paediatrician.

Questions

A 78-year-old woman with a 40-year history of chronic disabling rheumatoid arthritis gave a 2-month history of peripheral oedema and breathlessness. Her husband complained that her snoring was getting worse. She was on no medication apart from the occasional paracetamol.

On examination she was cachectic and pale. She had a symmetrical polyarthritis with deformities of her hands, feet and knees. There was oedema to her sacrum. Abdominal examination revealed hepatosplenomegaly and ascites. Her heart rate was 120 and she was in atrial fibrillation. She had a mitral systolic murmur and decreased breath sounds bilaterally.

The investigation results were:

- Chest X-ray – bilateral pleural effusions
- ECG – atrial fibrillation
- Haemoglobin 9.1 g/dL
- MCV 88 fL
- Urea – 11.0 mmol/L
- Creatinine 150 mmol/L
- Sodium 141 mmol/L
- Albumin 19 g/dl
- ALP 160 IU/L
- AST 180 IU/L
- Urine microscopy – hyaline casts
- Serum cholesterol 11.0 mmol/l
- 24-hour urine protein – 5.6 g

a. What is the cause of her current symptoms?
b. What is the cause of her increased snoring?
c. What is the underlying diagnosis?

Answers

a. Nephrotic syndrome (oedema and bilateral effusions). Her breathlessness is also due to fast atrial fibrillation and she probably had an element of congestive heart failure.

b. Macroglossia.

c. Secondary amyloidosis (longstanding rheumatoid arthritis). Amyloidosis in this case has caused nephrotic syndrome, hepatosplenomegaly, macroglossia and cardiac amyloidosis.

Discussion

Amyloidosis is the result of the deposition of amyloid protein in tissues. Many classifications exist related to the protein types involved but a simple clinical classification is primary and secondary. The primary form arises de nouveau and may be inherited. The secondary form is usually associated with chronic diseases, e.g. rheumatoid arthritis, ankylosing spondylitis, bronchiectasis, myeloma, Waldenström's macroglobulinaemia, non-Hodgkin's lymphoma.

Clinical features of amyloidosis include: macroglossia, purpura and bleeding, hepatosplenomegaly, lymphadenopathy, cardiac failure, nephrotic syndrome, gastrointestinal symptoms, e.g. diarrhoea, weakness and paraesthesiae, carpal tunnel syndrome. Diagnosis is made by biopsy of the rectum or gums. The hallmark is the finding of amorphous hyaline deposits, which show a green fluorescence under polarised light when stained with Congo Red. Treatment is symptomatic and that of the underlying disorder. Chemotherapy for primary amyloidosis does not affect outcome.

Nephrotic syndrome is the clinical syndrome of oedema, proteinuria, ($> 5\,g/d$) and a low plasma albumin ($< 20/dl$). It is more common in children than adults. Causes are:

1. Primary glomerulonephritis, e.g. minimal change, membranous.
2. Secondary glomerulonephritis, e.g. system lupus erythematosus, carcinoma bronchus lymphoma.
3. Infections, e.g. malaria, sphyllis, leprosy, hepatitis B.
4. Drugs, phenytoin, ACE-inhibitors, gold, penicillamine.
5. Bites, e.g. bee and wasp stings.
6. Metabolic conditions, e.g. diabetes mellitus, amyloidosis.

Renal function is usually normal but oliguric renal failure may occur rapidly. Plasma albumin and gammaglobulins are low but alpha II globulins, fibrinogen, factor VIII, platelets and cholesterol are high. This leads to susceptibility to infection and thrombosis and an increased incidence of ischaemic heart disease (hypercholesterolaemia). There may be secondary hyperaldosteronism.

Management includes that of the underlying condition as well as control of oedema (with diuretics, i.v. proteins), high-protein/low-salt diet, antibiotics for secondary infection and treatment of thrombosis. Prophylactic use of heparin to prevent thrombosis is controversial. Prognosis depends upon the underlying condition. In this case the prognosis is poor as this patient has developed multiple organ failure.

Questions

A 30-year-old man who had been married for 2 years visited his GP because he and his wife were unable to conceive. He was otherwise well and was taking no medication. His mother had maturity onset diabetes mellitus. He worked as a warehouse labourer and was finding physical work more difficult to perform. His GP noted he had bilateral ptosis and low-set ears. His heart rate was 66 b.p.m. and regular and his blood pressure was 110/60. His random blood glucose was 14.1 mmol/L but other blood tests were normal. His chest X-ray showed cardiomegaly and ECG 1° heart block.

a. Why was he finding his job more difficult?
b. What is the cause of his ECG abnormality?
c. What is the diagnosis?

Answers

a. Weakness and myotonia.
b. Cardiomyopathy.
c. Dystrophia myotonica.

Discussion

Dystrophia myotonica is an inherited autosomal dominant condition and is more common in males. The condition shows 'anticipation' in that its severity increases in succeeding generations.

Clinically there is myopathic facies (drooping mouth, transverse smile), ptosis (usually bilateral), frontal balding, low-set ears, wasting and weakness of facial muscles as well as shoulder and pelvic girdles and sternomastoids. There is myotonia (slow relaxation of muscle) demonstrated after shaking hands when the patient has difficulty letting go; this condition is exacerbated by cold and excitement. Percussion myotonia can be demonstrated by pressing muscles and making indentations, which then take some time to return to their normal form. This can be demonstrated on the tongue or neck muscles. Involvement of the tongue and pharynx by myotonia can cause slurring of the speech. Other features include:

1. **Subfertility** – testicular atrophy (as in this case). Less evidence exists regarding ovarian atrophy.
2. **Cardiomyopathy** – this can cause sudden death due to arrhythmias and also heart failure.
3. **Intellectual deterioration**.
4. **Diabetes mellitus**.
5. **Cataracts**.

Myotonia can be improved with phenytoin, procainamide and quinine. The progressive weakness causes disability for which there is no specific treatment.

Question

A 52-year-old retired policeman was admitted to Accident & Emergency (A & E) with a 2-hour history of central chest pain. He had a cardiac arrest shortly after admission and was resuscitated from ventricular fibrillation. His 12-lead ECG showed ST elevation in the anteroseptal leads. All baseline blood tests and chest X-ray were normal. He was given aspirin 150 mg stat and diamorphine 5 mg i.v. and a lignocaine infusion was commenced. He lived with his wife and 20-year-old son. He was wheelchair bound for the last 10 years due to multiple sclerosis, which was diagnosed 15 years previously. He smoked 20 cigarettes a day. He had an indwelling urinary catheter, and required help from his wife for most activities of daily living, including feeding. She gave up her job as an accountant 2 years previously to care for him.

When his condition was stabilised in A & E the medical registrar decided to admit him to a general medical ward and decided that further resuscitation was inappropriate but he was to receive symptomatic treatment. The medical registrar told his wife that his condition was critical.

Name two major omissions in the management of this man's condition.

Answers

a. Thombolysis was not given. This patient has no contraindication to thrombolysis and has presented within reasonable time of his myocardial infarction for treatment to be effective in reducing mortality and morbidity. Although chest trauma following resuscitation is a relative contraindication to thrombosis it was not present in this case.

b. In this case it is inappropriate for 'do not resuscitate' orders to be decided by the medical registrar alone. If possible, the patient should be involved in this discussion as should his wife, with his permission. In this case, the medical registrar is making a judgement on the patient's quality of life without involving him in circumstances where cardiopulmonary resuscitation (CPR) could be highly effective, as has already been demonstrated with this patient.

c. This patient should receive cardiac monitoring on the cardiac care unit for at least 24 hours rather than being sent to a general medical ward. Even if the patient rejects a further cardiac arrest procedure cardiac monitoring can still be useful to detect and treat pharmacologically any significant arrhythmias.

It is important that these treatment issues are discussed logically and with sensitivity with patients and their relatives.

Discussion

All hospitals should have a CPR policy. Several organisations (British Medical Association, British Geriatrics Society and the Royal College of Physicians) have issued guidelines on such policies. They include the need to involve patients in such discussions and where appropriate, with patient permission, their relatives. These discussions require skill in communication and sensitivity. Therefore knowing when and how to embark on such discussions requires further emphasis in medical training. The doctor must not only possess communication skills but also knowledge of the possible outcome following CPR. Certain conditions, e.g. carcinomatosis, renal failure and pneumonia are associated with poorer outcomes following CPR whereas cardiac conditions, e.g. myocardial infarction are more likely to respond to this treatment. There are other factors that may improve outcome, e.g. patient location, (cardiac care units are associated with better outcomes). Studies have shown that there is a 10% survival rate at 12 months following an in-hospital cardiac arrest.

There may be good reasons not to discuss CPR with patients, e.g. confused patients – if the patient refuses and if the procedure is deemed to be medically futile. It may be appropriate to involve the patient in discussion, particularly if the patient requests and initiates such discussion and also if the outcome may be favourable but the patient is deemed to have a poor quality of life. In this case, the patient may consider that he has a good quality of life. Also, his condition is suitable for CPR treatment. He should if possible be involved in discussion regarding his treatment but the timing of this will depend upon his medical condition and it may be useful to discuss the issues with his wife, who has retired from her profession to care for him. To exclude such a patient from these discussions and withhold such treatment when there is no evidence of medical futility is negligent.

Questions

A 52-year-old veterinary surgeon complained of a 4-day history of myalgia and malaise. He had had a severe headache for 1 day, nausea, vomiting and breathlessness. He had returned from a 1-month long Safari in Kenya 3 weeks previously. He was a smoker of 40 cigarettes a day. He had no past history or family history of note. On examination he was icteric, and had a conjunctival haemorrhage and a petechial rash on his trunk. His temperature was 38°C, pulse 100 b.p.m. and blood pressure 110/60. He had marked neck stiffness and there were bilateral basal crackles on chest auscultation. The results of investigations were:

- Haemoglobin 11 g/dL
- White cell count 15×10^9/L
- Platelets 400×10^9/L
- INR 1.2
- Bilirubin 50 µmol/L
- ALP 300 IU/L
- AST 216 IU/L
- Sodium 139 mmol/L
- Potassium 4.1 mmol/L
- Urea 21 mmol/L
- Creatinine 300 µmol/L
- Creatinine kinase normal
- Urine dip testing = protein +++ blood+ casts+
- Chest X-ray – pulmonary oedema
- ECG – widespread T-wave inversion

a. Which of the following statements are **true**?
   1. There is evidence of disseminated intravascular coagulation.
   2. He has had an acute myocardial infarction complicated by left ventricular failure.
   3. There is evidence of hepatitis.
   4. His cerebrospinal fluid (CSF) will show normal protein levels and a polymorphocytosis.
   5. He is at risk of a gastrointestinal haemorrhage.
b. What is the diagnosis?
c. What is the treatment?

Answers

a. 3 and 5 are true. There is no evidence of disseminated intravascular coagulation as there would be a thrombocytopenia, which is not present. The reason for his left ventricular failure and ECG appearance is a myocarditis, not a myocardial infarction. The CSF, which has a polymorphocytosis and normal protein, would be very unlikely to be caused by an infection – the most likely aetiology in this case. He has a haemorrhagic tendency as he has a petechial rash and a conjunctival haemorrhage, and therefore he is at risk of a gastrointestinal haemorrhage.

b. *Weil's disease (*leptospirosis icterohaemorrhagiae*).

c. Treatment is supportive, i.e the effect of myocarditis such as left ventricular failure in this case should be treated in the usual way and haemodialysis may become necessary if there is renal failure. Penicillin and tetracycline are effective in preventing leptospiral infection although there is little proven efficacy in established disease. However, antibiotics should be given.

Discussion

Leptospires are organisms that survive in water and wet environments and although they are carried by other animals without any illness, they are pathogenic to humans. The sero group that causes the most severe human illness is *leptospira icterohaemorrhagiae*. It is transmitted to man via infected water or the urine of infected animals. In Britain rats carry the organism and infected rats' urine can enter broken skin of humans, particularly if they swim in canals and walk fells etc. The infection occurs more commonly in men and there are about 50 reported cases per year in Britain. There is an occupational risk to farmers, veterinary surgeons and sewermen.

The incubation period is 10 days. The onset of the illness is sudden with fever, headaches, myalgia and conjunctival suffusion is common. There is a leptospiraemia and the organisms infiltrate organs producing an acute inflammatory reaction affecting capillaries, causing them to bleed. The haemorrhagic tendency results in a petechial haemorrhage, epistaxis and occasional gastrointestinal bleeding. Infiltration of other organs produces nephritis and renal failure, hepatitis, myocarditis and meningitis. The CSF shows a raised protein (0.5–1 g/L), lymphocytosis and a normal glucose. The blood count shows a polymorph leucocytosis. There is a mortality associated with the disease the peak of which occurs on the 14th day of the illness. Death is usually due to renal or cardiac failure.

The diagnosis is suggested by the clinical picture, occupational exposure and microbiological evidence. Leptospires can be cultured from the blood and urine and there is a rising antibody titre. Treatment is supportive and with penicillin as described above.

---

*P.S.A. Weil (1848–1916). German physician.

Questions

A 58-year-old woman complained of anorexia and early satiety. She had lost 2 stones in weight in 1 month. She felt weak and had noticed increasing difficulty in getting upstairs. On examination she was underweight and had a yellow/purple discoloration over her face and around her eyes. A similar rash was seen in areas on the dorsum of her hands. There was tenderness in the epigastrium and a fullness.

Results of investigations were as follows:

- Chest X-ray normal
- Haemoglobin 13.5 g/dL
- White cell count 4.1 × 10⁹/L
- ESR 68 mm/h
- Calcium 2.1 mmol/L
- ALP 300 IU/L
- AST 124 IU/L
- Albumin 31 g/L
- INR 1.4.

a. What is the most likely diagnosis?
b. List two investigations that would help you confirm the diagnosis.
c. What is the possible cause of the abnormal liver function tests?

Answers

a. Dermatomyositis.

b. Muscle enzymes (serum creatine phosphakinase and aldolase are grossly elevated) and electromyography (this shows a classical triad of short, small, polyphasic motive units, fibrillations, positive sharp waves and insertional irritability).

c. Liver metastases secondary to stomach carcinoma.

Discussion

When polymyositis is associated with a distinctive rash it is known as 'dermatomyositis'. It occurs more frequently in women (3:1) and the peak incidence is 40–50 years. There is a more acute form of dermatomyositis that occurs in children and is often fatal. There is an association with malignancy in about 10% of cases; the most frequently found carcinomas are: lung, stomach, breast and ovary. There is no evidence that treatment of the underlying malignancy alters the outcome of dermatomyositis.

Clinically the onset can be acute or chronic and the skin and muscle symptoms may occur separately or together. There is often general systemic upset with fever and malaise. There is weakness and tenderness usually of the proximal limb girdle muscles, especially the shoulders and with chronic disease fibrosis causes flexion deformities. The proximal myopathy is manifest when the patient has difficulty dressing and combing their hair, and getting up from a seated position and going upstairs. The classical skin rash is a purple or lilac discoloration occurring around the eyes in particular and also on the face. There is an erythematous dermatitis on the dorsum of the hands, particularly over the extensor surfaces of the joints. The thickened pads over the dorsal aspect of the proximal interphalangeal joints are known as *'Garrod pads'. There may be arteritic lesions around the nails and generalised telangectasia, particularly on the face and chest. There may be associated pulmonary fibrosis, cardiomyopathy and Sicca syndrome.

As well as an abnormal EMG as described earlier, the ESR is elevated as are the muscle enzymes; this is due to the inflammation and necrosis that occurs in the muscle. It is important to consider viral myositis, metabolic and endocrine causes in the differential diagnosis, as well as late onset muscular dystrophies.

Treatment is with high-dose prednisolone (60 mg daily) during the acute stage and azathioprine is also used as a steroid sparing agent. The prognosis depends upon the presence or absence of an underlying neoplasm. The natural history of the disease is with recurrent relapses and remissions over a 10–20-year period; the patient usually succumbs to respiratory and cardiac complications.

---

*A.E. Garrod (1857–1936). English physician.

Questions

A 70-year-old man complained of a 3-month history of backache and tiredness. He complained of breathlessness and palpitations on exertion accompanied by chest tightness. He did not have any gastrointestinal symptoms. He complained of polydipsia and had recurrent headaches. Investigations results were as follows:

- Haemoglobin 9.6 g/dL
- White cell count 4×10^9/L
- Platelets 180×10^9/L
- ESR 104 mm/h
- Albumin 30 g/L
- Calcium 2.8 mmol/L
- Urea 26 mmol/L
- Creatinine 300 μmol/L
- Random blood sugar 9.8 mmol/L.
- Blood film showed leuco-erythroblastic changes.

a. Explain his cardiovascular symptoms.
b. What is the most likely diagnosis?

Answers

a. He has angina that is being precipitated by his anaemia and also by the hyperviscosity syndrome which he has. He may also be having tachyarrhythmias that are precipitating the angina but the palpitations may in fact be a sinus tachycardia related to the anaemia. His breathlessness may be due to the anaemia or to reduced left ventricular function, which is caused by anaemia and poor myocardial oxygenation. It is also likely he has associated ischaemic heart disease. He has a headache probably related to hyperviscosity syndrome and his polydipsia is caused by hypercalcium (corrected calcium = 3.0 mmol/l). He is not diabetic, which is the other cause of polydipsia.

b. Multiple myeloma.

Discussion

Multiple myeloma or myelomatosis is more common in men over the age of 40 years. It is characterised by neoplastic proliferation of plasma cells in the bone marrow with lytic bone lesions and the production of monoclonal protein by the plasma cells, which is detected in the serum and urine. The paraprotein produced is IgG in 70% of cases and IgA in 30% of cases, and there are rare IgM and IgD as well as mixed cases. The abnormal protein detected in the urine consists of monoclonal light chains of the gammaglobulin molecules and precipitates out at 56°C and dissolves again at 100°C. This protein is known as '*Bence-Jones protein'. In 15% of cases Bence-Jones proteinuria is present without a serum paraprotein. The bone marrow usually shows increased plasma cells (usually > 30% of the bone marrow). A skeletal survey will show osteolytic areas often with an osteoblastic reaction and pathological fractures may occur. Hypercalcaemia is due to bone involvement and destruction. The peripheral blood usually shows a normochromic or a macrocytic anaemia and there is often neutropenia or thrombocytopenia due to bone marrow suppression. Rouleaux formation is common and plasma cells may appear in the peripheral blood. Leuco-erythroblastic changes can also be seen as in this case. A leuco-erythroblastic reaction is the appearance of erythroblasts as well as primitive white cells in the peripheral blood. This picture also occurs in the following conditions: myeloid leukaemia, bone marrow infiltration by carcinoma or fibrosis tuberculosis, myelosclerosis, severe haemorrhage, haemolysis, megaloblastic anaemia, lipidoses. In multiple myeloma there is often renal impairment (20% of cases) due to deposition of heavy gammaglobulin chains in the kidneys, hypercalcaemia or secondary amyloidosis involving the kidneys.

Clinical features consist of: bone pain; features due to anaemia; recurrent infection due to a suppressed immune system; hypercalcaemia producing polyuria, polydipsia, constipation, depression etc.; the hyperviscosity syndrome producing a bleeding tendency, cardiac failure, headache, features of secondary amyloidosis and a bleeding tendency due to thrombocytopenia.

Treatment consists of supportive therapy as well as chemotherapy. Melphalan or cyclophosphamide with or without prednisolone are often the drugs of choice. Poor prognostic features include: blood urea > 14 mmol/l, anaemia and hypoalbuminaemia.

*H. Bence-Jones (1814–1873). English physician.

Questions

A 25-year-old woman complained of a 6-week history of intermittent abdominal pain and diarrhoea. There was no history of passing blood or mucus per rectum (PR). She had had a similar episode 1 year previously, which resulted in an appendicectomy. She had lost 2 stones in weight in 12 months. Her mother had diabetes and her elder brother had chronic backache and psoriasis. On examination she looked pale and thin and there were several bruises on her legs. She had finger club-bing. Abdominal examination revealed tenderness in the right iliac fossa and increased bowel sounds. There was evidence of optic atrophy on fundoscopy but no other neurological signs. Blood tests revealed the following:

- Haemoglobin 10.1 g/dL
- White cell count 4×10^9/L
- MCV 90 fL
- Blood film diamorphic blood picture
- INR 1.6
- Albumin 28 g/L
- Sodium 140 mmol/L
- Potassium 3.0 mmol/L
- Urea 1.2 mmol/L
- Creatinine 120 μmol/L
- Calcium 1.7 mmol/L.

a. Explain her blood results.
b. What is the most likely diagnosis?
c. What is the cause of optic atrophy?
d. What is the most likely reason for her brother's backache?

Answers

a. The blood results and history, in particular weight loss, pallor and bruises point to malabsorption. She is hypoalbuminaemic and her raised INR is due to vitamin K deficiency caused by malabsorption. A low urea and potassium is consistent with malabsorption and the diamorphic blood pressure implies she is both iron and B_{12} deficient. She also has hypocalaemia (the corrected calcium being 1.94 mmol/l). Malabsorption has many causes and may be due to intestinal disease or a blind loop syndrome caused by bacterial overgrowth.

b. The most likely diagnosis is Crohn's disease as the history is recurrent and she had appendicectomy 1 year previously. There are also some clues in the family history in that her brother has psoriasis and backache, which is probably due to sacroiliitis and these are more common in patients with Crohn's disease and in their families. Coeliac disease is another possibility and a cause of malabsorption in this age group.

c. B_{12} deficiency causes optic atrophy. Other neurological consequences of B_{12} deficiency are: peripheral neuropathy, sub-acute combined degeneration of the spinal cord and dementia.

d. Sacroiliitis. Other associated diseases are: psoriasis, Reiter's syndrome and ankylosing spondylitis. HLA-B27 is more common in these conditions.

Discussion

Crohn's disease, also known as regional ileitis is a granulomatous inflammatory disorder of the intestine, which tends to occur in young adults at presentation. The small intestine is usually affected particularly the terminal ileum but any part of the gastrointestinal tract including the mouth and anus can be affected; the colon is affected in 20% of cases. The pathological process occurs in short lengths of bowel with normal bowel in between ('skip lesions'). There is chronic granulation of tissue with non-caseating granulomas and there is a regional lymphadenopathy.

Typical symptoms include abdominal pain that is colicky and there may be intestinal obstruction. Diarrhoea and features of malabsorption are common (in 50% of cases). There may be mouth ulcers and perianal sepsis (in 20% of cases). Other non-gastrointestinal features include:

- **Skin** – erythema nodosa, pyoderma gangrenosum
- **Arthritis**

- **Sacroiliitis**
- **Hepatic involvement** – gallstones, chronic active hepatitis, sclerosing cholangitis
- **Eyes** – iritis, episcleritis
- **Mouth** – stomatitis, ulcers
- **DVTs** – more common.

There is often tenderness in the right iliac fossa as the terminal ileum is most commonly involved. Frequently the patient has had an attack of the disease, has required an appendicectomy and the diagnosis is made histologically at this stage. The disease progresses with remissions and relapses. Surgery should be avoided if possible but often is required to relieve acute emergencies. Surgical procedures can be complicated by infections and fistulae. Management is usually with steroids and mesalasine to maintain remission.

---

*B. B. Crohn (Born 1884). American physician.

Questions

A 50-year-old woman complained of pruritus, anorexia and severe weight loss over a 12-month period. She had episodes of melaena 6 weeks prior to presentation. Her sister has thyroid disease and her mother had rheumatoid arthritis but there was no other family history of note. On examination she was thin, pale and icteric. There were scratch marks on her body. She had finger clubbing. There were bilateral basal crackles on chest auscultation and hepatosplenomegaly. Investigation results were as follows:

- Haemoglobin 7.1 g/dL
- MCV fL
- Bilirubin 100 μmol/L
- Alkaline phosphatase 1000 IU/L
- AST 106 IU/L
- Random blood sugar 6.1 mmol/L
- INR 1.7.

a. Which of the following statements are **true**?
   1. The cause of her melaena is most likely due to a peptic ulcer.
   2. Weight loss is due to an increased metabolic rate in this condition.
   3. Anti-neutrophil cytoplasmic antibodies (ANCA) will be positive.
   4. Treatment is symptomatic rather than curative.
   5. She most likely has associated pulmonary fibrosis.
b. What is the diagnosis?
c. What other diseases are associated with this condition name two?

Answers

a. 4 and 5 are true. It is unlikely she has a peptic ulcer and the most likely cause of her bleeding is oesophageal varices. Her weight loss is due to malabsorption and anti-mitochondrial antibodies are positive in 90% of cases in this condition. Anti-neutrophil cytoplasmic antibodies (ANCAs) are specific for Wegener's granulomatosis.

b. Primary biliary cirrhosis.

c. Systemic sclerosis, *Sjögren's syndrome, CRST syndrome, rheumatoid arthritis, †Hashimoto's thyroiditis, renal tubular acidosis, coeliac disease and dermatomyositis.

Discussion

Most cases of primary biliary cirrhosis occur in women (90%) and presentation is between 40 and 60 years of age. There is usually granulomatous changes around the bile ducts with progression to fibrosis and frank cirrhosis. This causes cholestatic jaundice, which is the common presenting feature resulting in pruritus. There is often skin pigmentation, finger clubbing and ultimately hepatosplenomegaly develops due to portal hypertension. Cholestatic jaundice results in an extreme elevation of alkaline phosphatase as in this case and a high level of bilirubin. The consequences of portal hypertension are oesophageal varices and their hemorrhage is often a terminal event. The other most common terminal event is hepatocellular failure. Treatment is with cholestyramine for the pruritus and fat-soluble vitamin supplements. Steroids and immunosuppressive therapy is not helpful.

---

*H.S. Sjögren; (Born 1899). Swedish ophthalmologist.
†H. Hashimoto (1881–1934). Japanese surgeon.

Abbreviation list

A&E	Accident and Emergency	GH	Growth Hormone
ACE	Angiotensin-Converting Enzyme	GP	General Practitioner
		Hb	Haemoglobin
ACTH	Adrenocorticotrophin Hormone	HLA	Histocompatibility Antigen
ADH	Antidiuretic Hormone	HOCM	Hypertrophic Obstructive Cardiomypathy
AIDS	Acquired Immune Deficiency Syndrome		
ALP	Alkaline Phosphatase	IgA	Immunoglobin A
ANCA	Anti-Neutrophil Cytoplasmic Antibodies	IM	Intramuscular
		INR	International Normalised Ratio
ASD	Atrial Septal Defect	LH	Luteinising hormone
ASH	Asymmetrical Septal Hypertrophy	MCV	Mean Cell Volume
		MRI	Magnetic Resonance Imaging
AST	Aspratate Aminotransferase		
		MVP	Mitral valve prolapse
BBB	Bundle Branch Block	p-ANCA	Peri-nuclear ANCA
c-ANCA	Cytoplasmic-ANCA	PR	Per Rectum
CPR	Cardiopulmonary Resuscitation	PTH	Parathyroid Hormome
		SABE	Subacute Bacterial Endocarditis
CSF	Cerebrospinal Fluid		
CT	Computerized Tomography	SAM	Systolic Anterior Movement (of the mitral valve)
DNA	Deoxyribonucleic Acid		
DVLA	Driving Vehicle Licensing Agency	SC	Subcutaneous
		TSH	Thyroid-Stimulating Hormone
DVT	Deep Vein Thrombosis		
EMG	Electromyogram	VSD	Ventricular Septal Defect
ESR	Erythrocyte Sedimentation Rate		
		VT	Ventricular Tachycardia
FVC	Forced Vital Capacity		
FEV	Forced Expiratory Volume		
FSH	Follicle Stimulating Hormone		

Index